Discussing Sexuality
A Guide for Health Practitioners

Michael W. Ross
MA, BS MPH DipTertEd PhD CPsychol FBPsS FRSH

National Centre in HIV Social Research
The University of New South Wales

Lorna D. Channon-Little
MSc PhD MAPsS MBPsS MISH

Department of Behavioural Science in Medicine
The University of Sydney

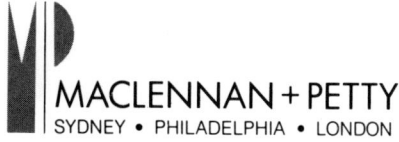

MACLENNAN + PETTY
SYDNEY • PHILADELPHIA • LONDON

For Peter and for Geoffrey

First published 1991
Reprinted 1993

MacLennan & Petty Pty Limited
80 Reserve Road, Artarmon NSW 2064, Australia

© 1991 MacLennan & Petty Pty Limited

All rights reserved including that of translation into other languages. No part of this book may be reproduced or transmitted in any form or by any means, electronic or mechanical, including photocopying, recording, or any information storage and retrieval system, without permission in writing from the publishers.

Copying for Educational Purposes

Where copies of part or the whole of this book are made under section 53B or section 53D of the Act, the law requires that records of such copying be kept and the copyright owner is entitled to claim payments.

National Library of Australia
Cataloguing-in-Publication data:

Ross, Michael W., 1952–
Discussing sexuality: a guide for health practitioners.

Includes index.
ISBN 0 86433 075 8.

1. Sex counseling. 2. Medical history taking.
3. Sex therapy. I. Channon-Little, Lorna D.
II. Title.

616.85830651

Printed and bound in Hong Kong

CONTENTS

Acknowledgements		vii
Foreword		ix
Preface		xi
1.	Introduction: Why take a sexual history? (MR)	1
2.	How to take a sexual history (MR)	6
3.	Taking a sexual history (LC–L)	17
4.	Sexual history taking for sexually transmissible diseases (MR)	34
5.	Sexual counselling (LC–L)	42
6.	Sexual counselling and treatment (LC–L)	48
7.	Reactions to STD infection and STD counselling (MR)	67
8.	Sexuality and preventive health care (MR)	88
9.	Sexuality and chronic illness (LC–L)	94
10.	Sexuality and drug-related history (MR)	100
11.	Pre- and post-test counselling for sexually transmissible diseases (MR)	104
12.	Legal and ethical considerations (MR & LC–L)	122
13.	Understanding and counselling the homosexual patient (MR)	131
Index		145

ACKNOWLEDGEMENTS

This book would not have been possible without help from a number of sources. Our particular thanks go to Karin Gylseth who prettied up manuscripts at a time when she was under considerable pressure from other work, and to Michael Drury who typed parts of the manuscript at short notice and was invaluable protection from disruption. Thanks are also due to Dr Norman Schum of Adelaide who did some sterling work persuading his local medical librarian to hunt down a particularly self-effacing reference, and to Bev Alcorn, of the Leichhardt Women's Health Centre who helped with the material about lesbian women.

Adis International Limited kindly consented to allow us to reproduce modified versions of several papers in *Patient Management* as sections of chapters. These include the following:

> Ross, M.W. Counselling the homosexual patient. *Patient Management*, 1983, 7(7), 117–123.
>
> Ross, M.W. Understanding the Homosexual patient. *Patient Management*, 1985, 9, 15–25.
>
> Ross, M.W., and Rosser, B.R.S. Pretest counselling for AIDS screening: a guide for the clinician. *Patient Management*, 1987, 11(7), 93–103.
>
> Ross, M.W., and Rosser, B.R.S. Counselling the patient with an STD. *Patient Management*, 1988, 17(8), 73–84.
>
> Ross, M.W. (1989) Principles of patient counselling. *Viral Therapy in General Practice*, 1989, 4, 1–3.

Finally, Dr Lyndon Wing of the Flinders University Medical School in Adelaide offered valuable advice and criticism on the chapter on sexuality and drugs, and his help was greatly appreciated. However, any errors in the text are solely the responsibility of the authors.

FOREWORD

It is now more than 30 years since I graduated in medicine. Today we live in a more interesting, more honest, and better equipped world. By comparison, that time of my graduation seems primitive and simple. Not only are we better able today to care for common conditions but, as this book sets out so well, we are better equipped and prepared to take good patient histories as part of offering better care.

The revolution in care in my professional lifetime has been enormous. We are watching the rapid decline in the mortality from ischaemic heart disease, we can now treat hypertension, we can (and do) prevent measles and poliomyelitis, we have eliminated smallpox, we understand better some nutritional principles, we have reduced markedly the incidence of tobacco use and we are reaping the rewards of some real gains in longevity and in years of quality life.

With all these gains, with the lessening of morbidity and mortality from traditional causes, we face new challenges and new imperatives. We now see a nation ready to address a multitude of lifestyle problems. For the first time we see real efforts being made to address the 'hidden' problem of alcohol abuse. And, in the same way we have come to realise that we must learn to address the challenge of sexually transmitted illness and of sexuality as a whole.

In my undergraduate days we taught sexuality about as badly as it could be done. We worked to a disease-oriented paradigm in disease-oriented institutional settings, so that we were 'taught' about sexuality in the cold, clinical, and detached atmosphere of the venereal diseases clinic. In those days it was not made easy for patients to give a history if that was likely to reveal inconvenient material, nor to express their anxieties or uncertainties, nor even to say what they thought about most matters affecting them. in the area of sexuality, this meant that communication was seldom encouraged, that conventional middle-class opinions concerning sexual mores held sway in the clinics as they did elsewhere in the hospitals, and that patients were invited only to speak and act as the 'grateful patient' stereotype allowed. As for counselling, it was given, if at all, by social workers or by psychiatrists – it just did not feature in the daily routine of the busy disease-treating doctor.

This book is different. It is part of the liberating new age, part of the empowering of a generation of students and practitioners, and of a community of people who will interact with those practitioners. The book guides us through each stage of taking a sexual history without uncertainty, embarrassment, and obfuscation in the process. Major question sets are laid out in boxes which are easy to read and to understand, while the text is simple and helpful. It discusses counselling in the same way and with the same benefits.

If much of medicine should be about empowerment of others this book will help to empower those lucky enough to read it. If much of medicine is about beneficence and justice then this book will promote those values. In the context of a profession in which ethical issues are becoming ever more important and dominant, this book is a significant ethical work which will assist in the promotion of the best ethical standards in medicine. For that, if for nothing else, we are deeply in debt to the authors.

PETER BAUME
Professor and Head
School of Community Medicine
University of New South Wales

Sydney, April 1991

PREFACE

We have always assumed that such a basic necessity as a book on sexual history taking and counselling would be not only readily available but also a common text in medical and nursing courses. Therefore our first response on being asked to write such a book was: why write another one? On attempting to find such texts we were surprised that there was little available, and what was available was either too specialised or too brief. Why was there so little material on such an important area?

As we are both teachers in medical schools as well as clinicians, and as we both teach human sexuality to undergraduate medical students, we were acutely aware of the need for adequate training in the area not only of human sexuality, but the practical skills necessary to take a history, make a diagnosis, formulate a treatment plan or make an appropriate referral. The advent of AIDS in the last decade together with increased public awareness and discussion of STDs such as herpes, gonorrhoea, chlamydia and syphilis, and pelvic inflammatory disease, in the last few years has meant that practitioners are more likely to be asked about STDs by their patients. Indeed, they are expected to be comfortable in discussing sexuality and STDs. However, our encounters with students and colleagues suggested that while most recognised the need, few had the skills necessary or were comfortable in taking a sexual history. This was not helped by the pressure of time in medical and nursing courses as a result of the increased complexity of medical science and technology. Nevertheless, we believe that the art of health practice is still as important as the science, particularly in an area as relatively neglected as sexuality.

In response to this perceived need we have written this book as a manual rather than as a text. In doing so we recognise that a substantial number of practitioners will have had no training in the area. Even more will have had only introductory exposure to human sexuality during their training. Therefore we have tried to combine the steps necessary to take a sexual history and make a diagnosis in as simple a form as possible giving the reasons for each step. This book is unashamedly aimed at the practitioner and does not attempt to create experts in sexual therapy. Rather, we are hoping to enhance the basic skills of practitioners in what has become an integral part of health practice. We hope that it will prove useful as a guide to sexual history taking and counselling for practitioners who feel the need to expand or refresh their clinical skills.

MICHAEL W. ROSS

LORNA D. CHANNON-LITTLE

Sydney, March 1991

CHAPTER 1

INTRODUCTION: WHY TAKE A SEXUAL HISTORY?

In the last decades, the subject of human sexuality has become the subject of debate in society and the media, and advertisements for condoms appear on prime-time television. The general public perceive it as a subject for proper debate and are probably better informed about this formerly taboo subject than at any time in western history. Sexuality has become an area in which there is better knowledge about what is common or uncommon, more concern about sexual performance, and greater willingness to seek help for sexual problems. In addition, the current prevalence of sexually transmissible diseases (STDs) including gonorrhoea, syphilis, genital herpes, human papilloma virus, chlamydia, and human immunodeficiency virus (HIV) has made it likely that most practitioners will be faced with the task of taking a sexual history.

Unfortunately, despite the increase in courses on sexuality in schools of medicine, nursing, social work and psychology (courses which range from the token to the thorough), many health practitioners are uncomfortable about or relatively untrained for taking sexual histories, diagnosis of sexual problems, or basic sexual counselling. Where more and more science and technology is being fitted into courses for health practitioners, areas such as learning to take a sexual history and diagnose sexual problems tend to be under-emphasised. Even if the basic skills exist, discomfort with the area of sexuality can discourage health practitioners from approaching the subject.[1]

The aim of this book is to provide a simple, straightforward guide for the health practitioner: the why, how, when and where of taking a sexual history, with sufficient detail of sexual dysfunctions and behaviours to be able to make a basic diagnosis and either carry out appropriate counselling or make a suitable referral. This book is divided into three sections: how to take a sexual history; how to diagnose sexual dysfunctions; and how to undertake basic sexual counselling.

Good reasons for needing to be able to take a sexual history

There are a number of good reasons why taking competent sexual histories are a necessary skill for the health practitioner. First, the medical practitioner or nurse is usually the point of first contact for the person with a sexual dysfunction or STD. Failure to treat the person or the presenting problem seriously and professionally will neither resolve the problem nor enhance the reputation of the practitioner.

Second, the health practitioner is **expected** by the patient or client to have some knowledge in the area. The great majority of people on the street believe that the general practitioner is the appropriate person to approach for problems with sexual dysfunctions, questions about sexuality, or STDs. While there are specialists from a number of professions who treat sexual dysfunction or STDs, it is expected that the general medical or nurse practitioner will at a minimum take a history, make a diagnosis, offer appropriate advice and either refer on or counsel the patient or client themselves.

Third, as we have already noted, sex has become a topic of discussion in newspapers and magazines, on radio and television, and even in social conversation. As a result, there is a greater concern about sexual problems, a greater awareness of the risks of STDs, and a greater willingness to ask questions or seek help. The incidence of asking about sexual matters has risen markedly since 1960, initially as a result of an increase in use of contraceptives such as the anovulant pill, and more recently spurred on by greater awareness of STDs (of which herpes and AIDS are probably the best known).

Fourth, the role of the general medical practitioner has changed. Now there is greater emphasis on primary prevention and health education, and a significant proportion of this relates to sexual matters. In women, the need for regular pap smears to detect cervical cancer, the need for choosing an appropriate contraceptive for her lifestyle and monitoring its use, screening for breast cancer (including mammography), and the possibility of pelvic inflammatory disease (PID) are all areas where the health practitioner should advise and educate the patient.

In men, as in women, the possibility of sub-clinical STD infection, and advice on appropriate prophylaxis such as condoms, or even in younger men advice on regular testicular examination for testicular cancer, are important aspects of preventive health care.

Good reasons why most health practitioners are not able to take a good sexual history

There are a number of good reasons why many health practitioners need guidance in taking a sexual history. First, the most difficult aspect in taking a sexual history is to avoid discomfort to both practitioner or patient. Comfort comes for the practitioner with both practice and a sense of control over the subject, and this comfort is communicated to the patient. The general lack of adequate instruction in sexuality, and lack of opportunities for practice in taking sexual histories which would normally desensitise the practitioner's discomfort, means that out in the community practitioners may need to enhance their skills before they are comfortable taking a sexual history.

Second, it may be that the practitioner is more embarrassed than the patient in taking a sexual history. If this is the case, then both will attempt to skirt around the subject and inadequate or inaccurate histories will be taken so that diagnosis will be subject to greater uncertainty or error. It will also ensure that in future, sexual problems are not raised.

Third, sexual dysfunctions and STDs are not uncommon and it will be rare for the practitioner in the community not to see one or two potential cases per year. We use the term 'potential' because if one doesn't ask about problems, they are usually not discovered. That does not mean they don't exist. For example, there is room for improvement in taking adequate histories of alcohol and drug use. The fact that adequate histories are not taken does not reduce the morbidity and mortality associated with substance use: if anything, it exacerbates it.

Health practitioners differ with regard to their estimates of the proportion of their patients who have sexual difficulties: surgeons estimate the proportion to be as low as 15%, psychiatrists suggest it may be as high as 70%. While these figures may also reflect the different types of patients seen, even if one in seven patients may have a sexual problem, the average practitioner may need to take at least one sexual history per day. Taking a sexual history and making a diagnosis, or providing sexual counselling, is a skill that the health practitioner should not be without.

There is some empirical evidence as to why medical practitioners have difficulties with sexual histories. Merrill and colleagues[2] identified three major reasons why practitioners fail to take adequate sex histories: embarrassment, a belief that a sex history is not relevant to the patient's chief complaint, and the fact that they are not adequately trained.

In a survey of senior medical students in the United States, Merrill and colleagues found that while 93% thought that knowledge of a patient's sexual practices was an important part of their patient's medical history, half felt poorly trained to take one, and a quarter felt embarrassed to ask the necessary questions.

A number of personal characteristics, they found, were related to difficulties in taking a medical history. Those who were most shy and socially anxious were most likely to feel embarrassment, while an unsympathetic view of patient's psychological problems was most closely related to the belief that the sex history was of little importance in understanding a patient's problem. The sense of not feeling adequately trained to take a sex history related most strongly to lower self-esteem. These data suggest that the difficulties in taking a sex history, while common, can be overcome with training and experience.

In addition to the prevalence of sexual dysfunctions, the AIDS epidemic has focussed attention on counselling associated with STDs. In some states, testing for HIV requires mandatory (by law) pre- and post-test counselling. It is often impractical to refer on to a counsellor unless one is associated with a specialist STD or AIDS clinic, so taking a sexual history and counselling will become a much more common requirement.

Finally, if particular health practitioners do not meet a need, then it is likely that patients will move to practices which do meet their needs. In urban areas, there is frequently a wide choice of practitioners and the inability to offer particular services or to deal comfortably with the full range of presenting problems may be one of a number of factors which lead people to shop around.

In summary, there are a number of compelling reasons why the health practitioner should be sufficiently competent to take **at minimum** a sexual history, if not to engage in basic sexual counselling. Even if the decision is to refer on, it is not possible to write an adequate referral without having taken a sexual history. And without a sexual history, it is not possible to determine whether the referral should be to a psychologist, psychiatrist, endocrinologist, neurologist, urologist, gynaecologist, marriage counsellor, general sex therapist, or whoever else may be appropriate.

If the presenting problem has STD as a possible diagnosis, then basic examination cannot take place without taking a sexual history to determine what sites should be investigated and the probable latency of infection to make differential diagnosis possible. The sexual history is a subset of a general medical history, and taking a medical history is probably the most basic and most essential skill of the health practitioner today. So it is not as if it is a totally new skill, nor one peripheral to modern clinical practice.

There are various opinions as to when to take a sexual history, but not on its importance. Lief[3] puts it this way:

> 'The vast number of problems that involve aspects of sexual functioning, the increase in the demand for services, and the expectation of patients that the health practitioner be competent and skilful in the management of sexual problems create a situation in which there is no real choice. The health practitioner must learn the basic skills of sex counselling or neglect a highly significant and important aspect of practice.'

References

1. Green, R. Taking a sexual history. In: Green, R. (ed.), *Human sexuality: a health practitioner's text* (2nd edn). Baltimore: Williams & Wilkins, 1979; 22–30.
2. Merrill, J.M, Laux, L.F and Thornby, J.I. Why doctors have difficulty with sex histories. *South Med J*, 1990: 83, 613–617.
3. Lief, H.I. Why sex education for health practitioners? In: Green, R. (ed.), *Human sexuality: a health practitioner's text* (2nd edn). Baltimore: Williams & Wilkins, 1979: 2–10.

CHAPTER 2

HOW TO TAKE A SEXUAL HISTORY

The sexual history should be seen as being a specific application of history taking, which follows the same principles and pattern as taking a general medical history. However, it also differs in four respects. First, it may engender embarrassment in both patient and practitioner. Second, it is likely, unless competently carried out and accepted by the patient, to lead to a greater proportion of false responses (usually false negatives) than any other form of medical history except possibly a psychiatric history. Third, because sexual anatomy and function are the subject of circumlocutions, particular care to establish that the language used is appropriate must be taken. And fourth, because of potential embarrassment and inaccurate responding, it is generally useful to explain the reasons necessary for taking a sexual history, particularly when the history is not being taken in direct response to a sexual presenting problem. For these reasons, a sexual history needs to be approached with more preparation than a general medical history.

Who to take a sexual history from?

Many authors suggest that a full sexual history should be taken from all patients. In a perfect system where time constraints, embarrassment on the part of practitioner and patient, and lack of general acceptance of sexuality as being an integral part of physical and psychosocial functioning, were not problems, this would be the approach of choice. However, because health practitioners are affected by all of the above to a greater or lesser extent, sensible utilisation of time and the need to maximise the detection of problems dictate that different approaches and indices of suspicion should apply. Four useful criteria on which to make decisions on how to approach a sexual history can be identified.

Age

Taking a sexual history for the very young will be considered inappropriate unless there is reason to believe that sexual activity may have occurred. If this is the case, then the issues in taking sexual histories from children require a totally different approach from taking a history in adults and should be referred to a child psychiatrist or psychologist. There are also legal considerations to be taken into account which are discussed in a later chapter.

At the other end of the spectrum, taking a sexual history from an aged widow or widower may also be difficult, both because of generally greater embarrassment in older people about sex, and because sexual activity may not be as frequent or as available in such a situation. On the other hand, sexual histories are probably mandatory for late adolescents and through to those in relationships (of whatever age). For those who are assumed to be sexually active, the issue should be raised.

Gender

There may be differences between men and women in sexual history taking. In the case of women, issues such as gynaecological functioning, contraception, and parity make it easier to raise questions of sexuality. In men this is more difficult, although it has been suggested that men are less reticent to discuss sexuality than women (such gender differences are probably disappearing). Where double standards of sexual behaviour occur, in which it is more acceptable for men than women to have multiple sexual contacts, or contacts outside relationships, then it is more likely that issues of STDs may need to be investigated in men. Conversely, such double standards also place a female partner at risk of infection from her spouse.

Context

The context of the consultation will also influence who is interviewed. The reason for the presentation, the pressure of time, the possibility of follow-up or of taking a fuller history at a later stage, whether the consultation is single or a joint one, and the perceived confidentiality of history and records will all be factors which may determine whether a screening or a full sexual history is taken. Whether one is the regular practitioner or is seeing the patient on a one-off basis may also be a consideration. In such cases, the practitioner may need to make a clinical decision about what priorities exist and in what order they should be approached.

Conservatism

The greatest barrier to taking a sexual history is conservatism on the part of both patient and practitioner. Clearly, taking a sexual history in someone with conservative views will be more difficult or will yield less cooperation or accuracy. However, we have been consistently surprised at how wrong we have been in our judgements of patients who we have expected to feel uncomfortable about having sexual issues raised. In general, the more conservative individuals are likely to have discussed sexual matters less, to have more questions about sexuality and sexual functioning, and to have greater difficulties with sexuality than more liberal individuals. Thus, while there may be concerns about raising the issue of sexual health with apparently conservative patients, there may be disproportionate advantages in doing so.

However, while there will be major individual differences in patients which may influence the decision to take a sexual history, or to influence whether such a history is a few screening questions or a full history, the practitioner should at some stage make an assessment of what the chance of sexual problems may be, and base this on information rather than guesswork.

When to take a sexual history?

Timing of the sexual history is important in its acceptance by the patient. Green[1] notes that the optimal time is not when the patient's initial visit has been prompted by influenza, nor on the third anniversary of the practitioner-patient relationship. The timing will depend on the reason why the practitioner needs to take a sexual history. Green argues that the sexual history should be taken when the full medical history is taken. However, we feel that the time to take a sexual history will depend on a number of factors, and that the most important of these is the **reason** the sexual history is taken. There are three reasons: screening, particular need for diagnosis, and specific sexual presenting problem.

Screening sexual history

The screening sexual history can be taken any time and is recommended for patients from whom a sexual history has never been taken, or patients who it is felt may not be receptive to having a full sexual history taken. It should be taken from all patients, although the timing is important. Where a **new** patient is being seen, the screening questions should be asked in the context of the general medical history. Where the patient has been seen previously, it is appropriate to add the screening questions into either relevant history, or into the preventive interview (discussed below).

Screening history in women: For women, the screening history should be associated with relevant areas of the medical history and follow from these. Such areas include history of pregnancy or childbearing, history of gynaecological problems, history of STDs or other genital infections, or history of pap smears and other investigations.

The sexual screening history in women consists of a minimum of four questions. These are:

1. Are you sexually active?
   (If 'No', When were you last sexually active?)
2. Do (or have you) had any discomfort or other problems during intercourse?
   (If 'Yes', Do these bother you?)
3. Have you had more than one sexual partner?
   (If 'Yes', How many and how long ago?)
4. Have you had any pain on passing water or unusual discharge from your genitals?
   (If 'Yes', take a history of this.)

Screening history in men: Much the same pattern occurs in taking a screening history in men. Again, it is appropriate for patients from whom a sexual history has never been taken, or patients who it is felt may not be receptive to having a full sexual history taken. However, opportunities for asking the screening questions are fewer in the case of men. Where a **new** patient is being seen, the questions should be asked following the history of any urological complaints or genital infections, bowel function, or relationship history. Where the patient has been seen previously, such questions may be asked in relevant areas of medical history taking or in preventive history sections as discussed further on in the book.

The screening history in men also consists of a minimum of four questions, virtually identical with those for women apart from the wording of the second question. The different form of the second question is designed to elicit problems associated with erectile dysfunction. The reworded question for men is:

2. Do you (or have you had) any difficulties or problems associated with sexual intercourse? (If 'Yes', Do these bother you?)

Reasons for asking screening questions: There are three reasons to ask these questions. The practitioner is seeking to communicate to the patient that sexual questions are acceptable and that he or she is open to sexual problems being brought up in the consultation. This acts as a provision of permission to discuss sexual questions or problems and confirms that the practitioner can be seen as competent to answer, treat or refer on sexual issues. The investment may pay off in the future when sexual issues arise.

Second, it provides an opportunity to address sexual problems if there are any existing ones, or to answer immediate questions. If sexual problems are apparent, then a fuller history is taken. And third, it alerts the practitioner to areas for further investigation or to the need for preventive education.

Taking a sexual history as part of a full medical history

Green[1] advocates that a full medical history should be taken on the first visit. Choice of the patient for whom such an approach might be appropriate will depend to some degree on the patient, the reason for the visit, and the confidence of the practitioner in initiating such an approach. It is worth quoting Green in full:

> 'The opening statement can be: "As your physician, I will be responsible for helping to maintain your health in all areas. Where your needs may call for more specialized care, I am prepared to refer you to a specialist colleague. One area of health which has been relatively neglected by physicians in the past is sexual health. It has become increasingly apparent that if we are to fulfil all our responsibilities to patients this important part of our lives must also receive attention. Therefore, I am going to ask you a number of questions about sexuality. Typically, there are certain issues which most frequently raise questions or cause concern. These include our sexual functioning, the types of sexual experiences we have, our sexual preferences, our sexual adjustment within or outside marriage, the sexual education of our children, the meaning of childhood sex play, teenage sexuality, and so forth. You should know that what we discuss is confidential, in the same way as the rest of your medical history." (p. 25).'

This full frontal approach to taking a sexual history may be appropriate for patients whom the practitioner believes are likely to be relatively comfortable with issues of sexuality and who are usually younger in age. However, such a full history may not always be the approach of choice for a number of reasons relating to the practitioner, the setting and the patient, although it is the fullest approach for the practitioner with time and experience and comfort to carry it out. The general sexual history in the absence of a specific sexual complaint should cover a number of areas. These include a history of puberty, commencement of sexual activity, sexual partners, sexual practices, current sexual relationships, history of sexual dysfunctions, history of STDs and drug history as well as details of parity, contraceptive or prophylactic practices where appropriate.

Taking a sexual history for specific presenting problems

Where the patient presents with a specific sexual problem, such as a possible STD, a sexual dysfunction or questions about sexual functioning, specific histories should be taken. These are covered in the following chapters since the nature of the problem will determine the approach, the questions and the issues which need to be covered to enable differential diagnoses to be set up. In such a case, the patient and the practitioner are in agreement on the need to take a sexual history and thus questions of embarrassment, inaccurate answers or dissimulation, or reasons for the history being taken are not so salient.

Taking a sexual history in relation to marital or emotional difficulties

Green[1] has argued that conflicts over sexuality can result in depression, anxiety, and alcohol and other drug abuse. Lief[2] notes that more people are troubled by marital and family relationships than by any other aspect of life such as work, money, recreation, or even addictive problems related to alcohol or drugs. We know that in three out of four cases of significant marital disharmony, there is a troublesome sexual problem. Such problems are most frequently those of sexual inadequacy and sexual incompatibility.

Where relationship issues or problems occur (and these may emerge only after sensitive probing by the practitioner when patients present with generalised psychosocial problems such as anxiety, depression, insomnia, tension or restlessness (questioning as to underlying sexual difficulties is essential. A general introduction followed by more specific queries is the approach of choice, with questions leading into the area such as:

1. How does your partner feel about your X (whatever the current problem is)?
2. Has X led to problems with how you relate to your partner, or s/he relates to you, for example emotionally and sexually?

3. (If 'Yes') In particular, what sexual problems have arisen or have been associated with X?

At this stage, the practitioner may move into taking a fuller sexual history as appropriate to the problem and as described in the following chapters. It is wise to have at the back of one's mind the possibility that sexual problems are commonly associated with relationship disharmony, either as a cause or as a consequence, and that this possibility should always be investigated.

Where to take a sexual history?

It would seem obvious that a sexual history should be taken in a clinical setting. However, because of the sensitivity of the issue, confidentiality should be assured. The history should not be taken with a third person present unless consent has explicitly been sought and given: having a receptionist or assistant coming in and out of a room can inhibit the process severely. Similarly, in casualty departments where cubicles are separated by curtains and where conversations several cubicles away can be accurately heard, a sexual history should not be attempted.

Nor should the sexual history be commenced when the patient is in stirrups or in any other vulnerable position. When the patient is likely to feel uncomfortable or threatened, discomfort, embarrassment and dissimulation are likely to be heightened. Similarly, closeness is related to comfort. Sitting either too close or too distant may convey opposite, but nevertheless potent, messages. A third issue relating to context is eye contact. Avoiding eye contact conveys embarrassment on the part of a participant. Conversely, in the context of a sexual history, seeking eye contact may convey other suggestions, such as voyeurism. It is wise to position oneself where eye contact can be both met and avoided without having choice in the matter.

Language in taking a sexual history

There are a number of simple rules about language when taking a sexual history, and about how to order the questions. This is perhaps the most difficult area for health practitioners once they have embarked on taking a sexual history. The difficulty is knowing whether the patient understands the medical or anatomical language used or, conversely, whether using colloquial language will offend.

Kinsey's Rule: This states that one should never invite a negative answer by asking people 'Have you ever ...'. In an area of embarrassment, most people will answer 'no' to everything but the most inescapably obvious behaviour. Kinsey and colleagues[3] always phrased their questions 'When was the last time you ...' or 'How often do you ...'. This provides evidence that the practitioner is accepting of sexual variation and that there are no value judgements being made. Never pose a question in such a way that a negative answer is the easiest response.

Goldman's Rule: This rule states that one should never assume that people know what words mean. Goldman and Goldman,[4] in their classic book on children's sexual thinking, provide a number of amusing examples of what people think particular anatomical and behavioural terms in common use among health practitioners mean. The uterus was thought to be a tunnel in Switzerland, a virgin was defined as a member of an ethnic group! Adults appear to have similar problems. It is embarrassing to recollect giving a lecture on AIDS to a final year high school class which focussed on risk behaviours. At the conclusion of the talk, one of the class asked what 'heterosexual' meant. On being asked, over a quarter of the class had no idea what the term, which was integral to the discussion, meant. It was assumed to be some abnormal behaviour. Other patients have commonly thought that 'homosexual behaviour' meant anal intercourse.

It is important to make sure that patients **understand** the terms that one is using, particularly, if there is any doubt, to get them to describe their understanding of what they mean. Anatomical charts are extremely useful and should be kept to hand if one is contemplating taking a sexual history, because circumlocutions abound and it is not uncommon for practitioner and patient to take the same term to mean something different.

Orwell's Rule: This is a related rule named after the English novelist George Orwell, who believed that one should never use a long word when one could use a short one. The more complex or latinate the word, the more likely it is to be misunderstood. Wherever possible, ascertain what the patient's vocabulary is and use it. On the other hand, to some patients, having the practitioner use colloquial or vulgar terms may offend or give the impression that professionalism is being sacrificed. A sensible middle approach is to describe acts ('Do you put your penis in her mouth?' rather than 'Do you engage in oral sex?'; 'Do you come?' rather than 'Do you achieve orgasm?') where there is less confusion.

In general, neutral colloquial terms are better than vulgar ones but it is essential to make sure that the terms are common in meaning. If either party is at all embarrassed, it is almost certain that confusion will be compounded.

Mitford's Rule: A cardinal rule of interviewing, described by the author Jessica Mitford, is (in the context of investigative journalism) to start with the kind questions, and leave the cruel ones until the end. In taking a sexual history, a similar principle applies. One should commence with the less confronting issues and put the patient at ease before asking more explicit and possibly embarrassing ones. The advantage of this is that it provides an opportunity for the practitioner to gain the confidence of the patient and to develop some degree of empathy. It is a mistake to commence with the most challenging issues: they should be built up to and left to the last if at all possible.

The issue of empathy

The major problem faced in taking a sexual history is that of embarrassment (on both sides) over discussing matters which are normally not talked about professionally. There are two ways to overcome this: through explanation, and through practice.

Explanation of reasons for sexual history

Traditionally, it has been uncommon for practitioners to explain the rationale for taking histories, although this is changing rapidly. It has become increasingly accepted that the patient is the practitioner's best ally in treatment and health maintenance One form of explanation suggested by Green[1] has already been described above. However, a less formal approach is to tell the patient that there are a number of things one needs to know in order to treat or to make a diagnosis. For example, partner numbers are a guide to risk for STDs, and necessary for contact tracing if infection is present. Sexual practices are a guide to what sites need to be investigated for STDs, and necessary to determine whether sexual dysfunctions are practice-specific. Sexual contexts are a guide to whether dysfunctions may be situation-specific. Simple explanations both provide a rationale for the questions and give the patient some feeling of being consulted and having some control over what may be a difficult process for them.

Practice

Green[1] suggests that the most eye-opening exercise in revealing sex history-taking distress is a practice session. Choose a professional colleague of the same sex. Ask questions about their sexual practices and areas of sexual conflict. If possible, audiotape or videotape the interview. In particular, listen and watch for hesitancies, vocal tone changes, and facial hints of interviewer or interviewee distress such as eye contact deflection, fidgeting, or other tension. It is most unlikely that practitioners will be able to take competent sexual histories without some practice to desensitise discomfort and provide feedback on what the person playing the patient finds creates discomfort.

Once this has been done, the second step is to role-play a particular sexual problem, and to alternate the roles of patient and practitioner several times. This should be repeated using a colleague of the opposite sex, or partner or spouse. Because of the sensitive nature of a sexual history, feedback is critical (far more so than in any other area of medical or psychological history taking) to minimise discomfort for both practitioner and patient. Our experience is that often practitioners are more embarrassed than patients when sexual issues are raised. This is not surprising: in general, medical and other health practitioners are among the more socially conservative in the population. The interviewer who is ill at ease discussing sexuality communicates this to the patient. This has the function of inhibiting patient communication and shaping or biasing patient responses.

Discomfort

Because professional people spend a longer time preparing or competing for tertiary admission and in their professional studies, for some the experience of life and sexuality in late adolescence and early adulthood may not be as extensive or may occur later than in other sectors of the population. Class differences in sexual behaviour have also been consistently noted from the studies of Kinsey and colleagues,[3,5] with working class people starting their sexual experience earlier and having a greater variety of partners. On the other hand, the range of sexual practices is greater among professional people.

The consequence of this is to allow moral values to enter, either subtly (through vocal tone or expression, or facial expression) or overtly, into the sexual history-taking procedure. Our private attitudes may favour the lifestyle of one person over another. However, this attitude does not belong in the clinical interview or in responsible patient management. That is not to say that when advising on preventive aspects of sexual health, risks or consequences of particular practices should be avoided: quite the opposite. However, one's private belief about termination of pregnancy, marital monogamy or homosexuality is irrelevant to the conduct of the fact-finding sexual history. Even if practitioner discomfort is such as to make referral a responsible option, such a referral should be accompanied by a competent letter of referral setting out the relevant findings and if possible a formulation of the problem.

In summary, taking a sexual history should be an integral part of the skills of health practitioners. However, it is usually not taught or taught with severe time restrictions or minimal practice. Because of the discomfort felt by many practitioners and patients about discussing sexuality, taking a sexual history cannot (like almost any other clinical exercise) be taught solely from a book. In addition to the guide-lines above, **practice** (which includes feedback from colleagues and partners) is essential in adding sensitivity and polish into an area of history taking which requires it more than almost any other of clinical practice.

References

1. Green, R. Taking a sexual history. In: Green, R. (ed.), *Human sexuality: a health practitioner's text*. (2nd edn). Baltimore: Williams & Wilkins, 1979: 22–30.
2. Lief, H.I. Why sex education for health practitioners? In: Green, R. (ed.) *Human Sexuality: a health practitioner's text*, (2nd edn). Baltimore: Williams & Wilkins, 1979: 2–10.
3. Kinsey, A.C, Pomeroy, W.B and Martin, C.E. .*Sexual behaviour in the human male*. Philadelphia: W.B. Saunders, 1948.
4. Goldman, R, and Goldman, J. *Children's Sexual Thinking*. London: Routledge and Kegan Paul, 1984.
5. Kinsey, A.C, Pomeroy, W.B, Martin, C.E and Gebhard, P.H. *Sexual behaviour in the human female*. Philadelphia: W.B. Saunders, 1953.

CHAPTER 3

TAKING A SEXUAL HISTORY

Before you begin

Make sure that the physical setting of your rooms conveys a feeling of comfort and ease. Many people find that for sexual counselling and history-taking it is often best to set up two similar chairs at right angles. This avoids the confrontational eye contact you can get if you have a desk between you and the patient and allows him or her to look away if wished. It's also less authoritarian.

Plain speaking

It's important to use simple terms. Some people suggest that it's a good idea to ask the patient what terms are used for different body parts. It's simpler to lay down your own rules so that they are the same for every patient, however. Use proper medical terms such as 'penis' and 'vagina' and explain them with models or drawings if needed. Check that the patient understands what you mean if you use any words which are not often encountered in everyday speech.

Taking a sexual history from a woman

Getting started

A simple question like 'Tell me what brings you here' may well be all the lead in you need. You may well be able to keep the narrative going by using nods, an attentive listening posture and encouraging noises. Leave the patient as much time as she needs to tell her story before you go on to take a formal history. Be alert for signs of embarrassment or discomfort.

Remember, in cases presenting with sexual dysfunction the patient has already made two major steps forward, deciding that there is a problem and seeking help, but she may still feel uncertain now that she is actually in a formal consultation.

Beginning the formal history

In any interview situation, it's a good idea to begin with areas which are non-threatening. Most women feel relatively relaxed talking about their menstrual history, and this is a logical chronological place to start. Box 3A gives you some ideas for questions. Question 3 is particularly important as it introduces the idea that the interview will be about feelings as well as facts.

BOX 3A

Questions to ask about menstruation

1. How old were you when your periods started?
2. Were you prepared for the start of your periods? (Probes: parents, schools, peers.)
3. How did your parents express their feelings and thoughts about sex? (Probes: Expressions of affection? Attitudes to sexuality?)
4. Can you remember how you felt at the time?
5. Have you ever had any difficulties with your periods? (Probes: premenstrual tension, irregularity, heavy bleeding, pains or cramps, other.)
6. If you are still having periods, how regular are they?
7. If you are not still having periods, can you tell me what happened before they finally stopped?

Watch body language at this time. Is your patient sitting in a relaxed posture? Does her voice convey anxiety or discomfort?

Obstetric history

This may seem a little out of place, but again it's a fairly safe topic. Box 3B outlines some questions to use here.

It's particularly important at this stage to convey a non-judgemental attitude to the woman who reveals that she has had one or more abortions. One practitioner put her foot in it firmly when she responded to a patient's report of an abortion by saying, 'Oh, you poor thing. That must have made you feel terrible'. The patient, perhaps as a defensive rationalisation, took the attitude that the pregnancy was a reassurance that all was well with her reproductive system and was very angry that she was being pushed into feeling guilty.

BOX 3B

Questions to ask about pregnancies

1. How many times have you been pregnant?
2. Can you tell me what happened with each pregnancy?
   (Probes: medical problems, planned or unplanned pregnancy, miscarriages, abortions.)

Intercourse history

By this time the patient will have got the idea that sexual matters are being discussed in a sensible and professional manner. Again, you need to be sensitive to verbal and non-verbal indications of tension or embarrassment.

Don't make the assumption that your patient first experienced intercourse in the context of a long term relationship, nor that all her sexual relationships have been heterosexual.

Box 3C gives some sample questions.

BOX 3C

Questions to ask about intercourse history

1. Tell me what happened the first time you had sexual intercourse.
2. How did you feel about it at the time?
   (Probes: Worries about pregnancy, worries about sexual competence, guilt, emotional involvement with partner.)
3. What were your physical responses?
   (Probes: Lubrication, orgasm.)
4. Tell me about experiences after that.

Current sexual relationship

In this section you will build up a picture of what is happening in the current relationship — how it began, what emotional and sexual factors are operating, what the couple's power structure is like.

If the patient is involved in more than one relationship remember that her sexual and emotional responses may be quite dissimilar with the different partners. Again, a non-judgemental attitude is essential.

In cases of sexual dysfunction at least one partner views the dysfunction as a problem. You need to find out which one and what effect it has had on them both.

Box 3D suggests some lead-in questions.

BOX 3D

Questions on her current sexual relationship

1. How did you meet your current partner?
   (Probes: Where? How long ago? What attracted you to him/her? Dating pattern?)

2. What happened physically in the early stages of the relationship?
   (Probes: How did the patient respond to kissing? cuddling? petting?)

3. What happened when you first had intercourse with your partner?
   (Probes: What led up to it? Situation? Who decided on intercourse? Patient's emotional response? Her sexual response? Contraception?)

4. What sort of person is your partner?
   (Probes: Good points? Bad points?)

5. How is the relationship going?
   (Probes: Good things? Bad things?)

Current sexual behaviours

This section of the history gives you a clear picture of the patient's current sexual practices.

Don't be surprised that a small percentage of women will tell you that they simply don't know whether or not they have ever had an orgasm.

The section on infertility is particularly important. The mechanisation of timing and positions for intercourse when couples are trying to conceive can ruin a previously happy sexual relationship (see chapter six).

Box 3E offers some questions.

BOX 3E

Questions on current sexual behaviours

1. Tell me about your current sexual intercourse pattern.
   (Probes: partners, emotional involvement with partners.)
2. About how often do you have intercourse?
   (Probes: Does this suit you? Your partner?)
3. About how often do you reach a climax when making love? If you do not climax, do you fake it? What are your reasons for that?
4. Do you have any problems with lubrication?
5. Are you using any form of contraception currently?
   (Probes: Satisfactoriness of the method for the woman, her partner?)
6. Have you had any problems getting pregnant?
   (Probes: Her problem? Her partner's problem? Investigations? Interventions, pharmalogical and surgical? Effects on sexual and emotional relationship?)
7. Have you ever masturbated? Do you do so now?

Older women

About 10% of women of menopausal age or older suffer vaginal atrophy, which can result in painful intercourse. Some women avoid sexual intercourse because of this and the partner may feel rejected and sexually frustrated.

Another cause of painful intercourse at this time of life is vaginal dryness: it may simply take longer for the woman to become sexually aroused and lubricate. Sometimes there is little lubrication in spite of arousal.

A high proportion of women presenting at menopause clinics show loss of libido[1] and this can also have disruptive effects on the relationship. However, for other women the removal of the risk of pregnancy has the positive effect of allowing them to relax and enjoy intercourse more. Whenever you encounter loss of libido, be alert for the possibility of depression as a contributing factor.

Box 3F suggests some questions to ask older women.

BOX 3F

Questions to ask older women

1. Has the frequency with which you have intercourse changed over the past few years? Can you think of any reasons for this?

2. Has your enjoyment of sexual intercourse changed since your menopause?
   (Probes: Increased? Decreased? How does your partner feel about this?)

3. Have you experienced painful intercourse of late?
   (Probes: Lubrication? Arousal level?)

4. Has your partner changed in any way as far as sex is concerned?

Lesbian and bisexual women

Most lesbian and bisexual women will present to a Women's Health Centre or a lesbian practitioner if they have the choice. Sometimes that choice is simply not available. If you have little knowledge of lesbian sexuality, we suggest you consult JoAnn Loulan's book.[2] It is not only sensible and explicit, but has a good bibliography.

Sexual dysfunction

Sexual problems may be organic in origin, but the majority are psychogenic. Box 3G lists possible organic causes. Of course, it's essential to screen for organic factors. Even if a clear-cut organic cause is found, the sexual dysfunction is likely to have ramifications in terms of the response of the woman and her partner to the problem. Counselling may be needed, especially if the problem cannot be fixed.

Anorgasmia

This is probably women's most common complaint. They make love with a partner they care about, become sexually aroused but do not reach a climax. The problem may be primary, where the woman has never had an orgasm, or secondary, where failure to reach orgasm develops later. (The word 'failure' is a tell-tale here. Either or both partners may perceive the lack of orgasm as a failure situation.)

BOX 3G

Some possible organic causes of dysfunction

1. Acute or ongoing illness, especially if there is fever or lethargy.
2. Cardiovascular disease — there is a popular myth that sex is dangerous after infarct.
3. Endocrine disorders such as Addisons disease.
4. Diabetes — some women report loss of libido and anorgasmia.
5. Chronic illness such as arthritis, emphysema, multiple sclerosis, chronic benign pain, etc. These are dealt with more fully in chapter nine.

BOX 3H

Questions to ask about anorgasmia

1. How do you and your partner initiate sexual intercourse?
2. Do you usually welcome the idea? How do you respond?
3. What happens during foreplay?
   (Probes: Touching? Where? Time spent? Variety?)
4. How do you feel sexually during foreplay?
   (Probes: Sexual responsiveness of body parts such as nipples and vagina? Level of relaxation?)
5. Do you begin to lubricate during foreplay?
6. (For heterosexual relationships) how do you feel when your partner inserts his penis?
   (Probes: Sexually? Emotionally?)
7. How do you feel after intercourse?
   (Probes: Relaxation level? Sexual satisfaction? Abdominal discomfort? Emotional closeness to partner?)
8. Have you ever masturbated? Do you now?
   (Probes: Climax? Any guilt feelings? Other feelings?)

Some women in this situation feel sexually dissatisfied and may suffer abdominal pain resulting from vasocongestion. Another group is typified by the patient who responded to a question about whether she was sexually satisfied after intercourse. 'I feel great. **He's** the one who gets upset.' Remember that almost every woman from time to time experiences intercourse which does not lead to orgasm — what Alex Comfort[3] refers to as the 'wrong man at the wrong time' scenario. This is **not** anorgasmia.

Some questions to ask about anorgasmia appear in box 3H (see p 23).

General sexual dysfunction

Here the woman experiences little or no response to sexual stimulation. She does not feel aroused and the physiological responses — abdominal vasocongestion, ballooning of the vagina with the formation of the orgasmic platform, lubrication — are all absent. Sexual intercourse is likely at best to be uncomfortable and unrewarding and at worst downright distasteful.

Some women seem not to mind their unresponsiveness and here presentation is usually a result of the partner's initiative. Other women find the condition most distressing. The impact on the couple varies greatly. It is most disruptive when the woman avoids the initiation of intercourse by such means as going to bed at a different time to the partner or the traditional 'headache'.

Anxiety may be a causal or contributing factor. Assess it by direct questioning and observation of such non-verbal cues as body language and tone of voice. Anger and hostility to the partner may also be implicated.

This is an area where the woman's early experiences with sexuality are particularly important. She may well have learned her lack of response in a family which had repressive and puritanical attitudes towards sexual matters. Any unpleasant sexual experiences such as rape may also contribute.

Unlike erectile dysfunction in the male, neither anorgasmia nor general sexual dysfunction preclude intercourse. The impact on both partners of a sexually unenthusiastic and unpleasured woman needs to be considered.

Box 3I contains some questions to ask in cases of general sexual dysfunction.

BOX 3I

Some questions in generalised sexual dysfunction

1. How did your parents express affection?
   (Probes: To each other? To her?)

2. What did your parents teach you about sex when you were a teenager?
   (Probes: Readiness to discuss? General attitude to her sexuality?)

3. Have you had any unpleasant experiences with sex?
   (Probes: Rape? Exhibitionist? Dyspareunia?)

4. How do you feel when you or your partner starts to make love?
   (Probes: Angry? Fear of failure? Resignation or indifference?)

5. How does your partner feel about your responses?

6. Is there anything in your current situation that makes sex unpleasant or difficult for you?
   (Probes: Partner's hygiene? Circumcision? Possible interruptions? Tiredness?)

Vaginismus

In vaginismus the woman experiences an involuntary spasm of the muscles in the vaginal region. This makes intercourse painful or impossible.

It is difficult to assess the incidence in the population, but studies of presentations to specialist clinics suggest that it is seen in about one in ten presentations.[4,5]

In the vast majority of cases the causes are psychological. For about one in ten the problem has an organic cause and hence a physical examination is imperative.

History-taking should focus strongly on the relationship because both partners' responses may be involved in perpetuating the problem. It's also a good idea (as in most situations) to find out why the patient is presenting at this particular time. It may be that there has been a deterioration in the relationship and she feels that she has been blamed for the problems and pressurised into coming.

Some possible questions are shown in box 3J.

The physical examination which follows should be carried out as gently as possible, with the realisation that the patient probably has many anxieties about being touched in the vaginal area.

> **BOX 3J**
>
> ### Questions to ask when vaginismus is a problem
>
> 1. What happens to you when your partner initiates an intercourse situation?
>   (Probes: Arousal? Lubrication? Response of vaginal muscles? Any penetration? Her feelings?)
> 2. How does your partner react when your muscles go into spasm?
>   (Probes: Frustration? Anger?)
> 3. Has your partner reduced the frequency of attempted intercourse?
> 4. Have you ever been able to have intercourse?
>   (Probes: Partner? Situation?)
> 5. If you were once able to have intercourse, can you think of anything that might have caused the change?
> 6. What sort of things did your parents tell you about sex when you were a teenager?
>   (Probes: Puritanical attitudes? Warnings about pregnancy?)
> 7. Have you had any unpleasant sexual experiences?
>   (Probes: Rape? Childhood sexual abuse? Partner wishing uncomfortable, painful or distasteful practices? Ambivalent feelings about partner or situation?)

Finishing up

Your aim here is to make sure that the patient leaves your office feeling more relaxed and confident than she did when she arrived.

Before you finish the interview, ask if there are any areas that have not been covered. Then ask if she has any questions to ask you.

The final step is to make sure, even if you have given a referral to a sex counsellor, that the door is left open for further consultations. It is very easy for a patient to feel that she has somehow done or said the wrong thing if the consultation is obviously an end to the matter as far as you are concerned. Many patients find it very difficult to talk about sexual matters and feel betrayed and abandoned if they are simply referred elsewhere with no expression of interest in the outcome.

Taking a sexual history from a man

Getting started

It's less easy to begin a sexual history with a male patient as there is no equivalent of the 'safe' female topic of menstruation. When the presenting problem is clearly a sexual difficulty, there is an obvious place to start. In other situations, for example chronic illness, it's best to start with a 'normalising' statement. 'Your sexual functioning is just as important as, say, your stomach function. I always ask patients a little bit about how things are going sexually'.

Early sexual history

The first step is to see what kinds of attitudes and behaviours prevailed at home, school and so on. Did he feel free to discuss sexual matters with one or both parents? How did parents express affection to him? To each other?

Then, move on to his own sexuality. Again, a 'normalising' question can help. 'Many men's first experience of their own sexuality is a wet dream. You wake up with a damp, sticky feeling on your pyjama bottoms. Can you remember when that first started happening to you?' (If you ask whether it happened, the patient is much more likely to deny that it did.)

Masturbation is another topic that benefits from the normalisation approach. 'Most men masturbate at some time in their lives.' Check that the term 'masturbation' is understood.

Then move on to early experiences of intercourse. Pay particular attention to matters of timing. Many a man who becomes a premature ejaculator shows a clear history of **learning** the behaviour. Rapid sessions in situations such as a parked car or the parental home put a premium on coming quickly.

Current sexual relationships

The next area to consider is the person's current sexual relationship (or relationships). Do not assume that a person's sexual partners are all of the same sex. It is imperative to ask about gay relationships directly, as many people are less willing to volunteer information about same-sex contacts.

The overall aim in this section is to find out what is happening and how satisfactory it is to the people involved.

Box 3K outlines the areas.

---- BOX 3K ----

Questions on current sexual relationships

1. About how often do you have sexual intercourse?
   (Probes: How well does that suit you? Your partner(s)?)
2. Do you have any problems getting or maintaining an erection?
   (Probes: For how long? Partner? Situation? Anxiety about it?)
3. After you insert your penis, about how long does it take before you ejaculate?
   (Probes: Satisfaction to self? Satisfaction to partner?)
4. How enjoyable do you think your partner finds sexual intercourse?
   (Probes: Enjoyment of foreplay? Orgasm?)
5. Do you currently masturbate? About how often?
6. What form of contraception do you currently use?
7. What sort of person is your partner?
   (Probes: Dominance in the relationship? Enjoyment of physical affection?)
8. If the two of you are having any sexual difficulties, how do you respond?
   (Probes: Own response? Partner's response? Recriminations?)
9. Have you had any homosexual contacts?
   (Probes: How many? Satisfactoriness? Emotional responses?)

Sexual dysfunction

The most common male problems are erectile dysfunction, premature ejaculation and, rather more rarely, retarded ejaculation.

There is a greater pressure on males than females to perform sexually. A woman can always fake an orgasm, but a man cannot fake an erection. Not only are male difficulties more obvious and more likely to make intercourse impossible, but there is a greater social expectation of male sexual competence. As we said earlier, female anorgasmia may be perceived as a failure on the part of her male partner.

When intercourse difficulties clearly relate to a man's problems, he may have feelings of inferiority, guilt and inadequacy. His partner may respond with belittling comments, anger, a feeling that she is sexually unattractive and so on.

Erectile dysfunction

The plain truth of the matter is that most men will fizz once or more in their sexual lives. Problems arise when the man feels traumatised by the event and worries about a recurrence. Anxiety and tension make it less likely that he will get a functional erection.

The distinction between primary erectile dysfunction (the man has never achieved an erection sufficient to penetrate vagina or anus) and secondary dysfunction, where the difficulty arises after previously adequate erectile capacity, is not of any great value.

The main differential diagnosis that needs to be made is between organically-based and psychogenic dysfunction. Problems related to medication, disease processes such as diabetic neuropathy, neurological damage and so on need to be screened out. Even if a clear organic cause is found, the patient and his partner may still be in need of counselling.

There is a double-edged sword here. Of course, no physician would want to miss an organic diagnosis. On the other hand, both the patient and his partner may have a vested interest in finding an organic cause. The patient can then say that it is not his fault. The partner need not feel that he or she is a sexually-unattractive package. Also, over-assiduous searching for underlying pathology will only encourage the belief that nothing can be done.

The questions in Box 3L will help you establish whether or not the dysfunction is psychogenic. If a man can get a satisfactory erection in some circumstances (say, with one partner rather than another) the dysfunction may reasonably be viewed as a psychological problem and treated by behavioural methods (see chapter six).

Premature ejaculation

There are different definitions of premature ejaculation — from time elapsed between intromission and orgasm, the number of thrusts before the man comes or Masters and Johnson's[6] operational definition of sufficient time after intromission for a female partner to reach orgasm on fifty percent of occasions. The last suggestion seems to disregard the fact that many women are anorgasmic with intercourse alone and to regard premature ejaculation as a problem of heterosexuals only.

Perhaps the only working definition is that the man and his partner wish he could last longer.

The most useful knowledge to be armed with is the Kinsey Report[7] finding that about three quarters of the men in their sample reported

> **BOX 3L**
>
> ### Questions to ask in erectile dysfunction
>
> 1. Do you ever get erections?
>   (Probes: During the night? When you wake up? When masturbating? With erotic magazines, pictures, videos, etc.?)
> 2. Describe what happens when you start to make love?
>   (Probes: Who initiates it? How? Anxiety? Anger? Fantasies?)
> 3. Do you begin to get an erection at all? What happens to it?
> 4. Does the problem apply to all your sexual partners?
>   (Probes: Homosexual partners? Workers in the sex industry? Extramarital relationships?)
> 5. Are you on any medications?
> 6. Do you usually drink alcohol before sexual intercourse?
> 7. Do you suffer from any long-term illness? (See chapter nine for some chronic illnesses that may affect sexual function.)
> 8. How does your partner react to the problem?

ejaculating within two minutes of intromission. You can turn a self-styled premature ejaculator into a normal male with a single sentence.

Nonetheless, many men and their partners would like some help in prolonging intercourse time. Box 3M gives guidelines for interviewing and chapter six outlines therapeutic approaches.

Retarded ejaculation

Retarded ejaculation is when a man either takes a very prolonged period of time from intromission to ejaculation or fails to ejaculate at all. The cause may be organic, the result of medication or psychological.

Anti-depressives, anti-psychotics, narcotics, the benzodiazipines are among the many drugs which cause retarded ejaculation in some patients. Often the man will notice a connection between his medication and retarded ejaculation, do a cost-benefit analysis and perhaps take himself off the drug.

Organic causes of retarded ejaculation include diabetic neuropathy, multiple sclerosis, neurological damage and so on. The characteristic

---
BOX 3M

Questions to ask in premature ejaculation

1. Can you tell me about your early experiences of masturbation?
   (Probes: Secrecy? Need for speed? Emotional responses?)
2. Now, think back to your early experiences with sex, what were they like?
   (Probes: Partners? Situations? Emotional responses? Need for rapid ejaculation? Sex industry workers?)
3. About how long do you spend in foreplay? Do you ever have to ask your partner to stop touching your penis because you are nearing ejaculation?
4. About how long does it take from the time you insert your penis to the time you ejaculate?
   (Probes: Satisfaction to self? Satisfaction to partner?)
5. About how long would you like to last before ejaculation?
   (Probe: Would your partner tend to reach orgasm in that time?)
6. Is there any way your partner can reach orgasm after you have ejaculated?
7. Has this pattern of relatively early ejaculation always been true of you?
   (Probes: Other partners? Homosexual contacts?)
---

feature of organically based retarded ejaculation is that the problem is seen in all sexual circumstances. Careful, specific questioning is needed to establish this fact.

Psychogenic retarded ejaculation can also have a variety of causes. Sexual guilt, a traumatising sexual experience and dislike of a particular sexual partner are the most common. A very full history of past and current sexual experiences may furnish clues here.

While some partners of men who show retarded ejaculation may initially be delighted by their discovery of a sexual athlete, they tend rapidly to find the phenomenon rather dull and, given a man who feels he must go on until he ejaculates, even painful.

Some men with retarded ejaculation fake orgasm to avoid the embarrassment of admitting their problem. Retarded ejaculation should always be considered a possibility when investigating infertility.

Box 3N outlines some areas to cover.

BOX 3N

Questions to ask in retarded ejaculation

1. About how long does it take you to come after you have inserted your penis?

2. Do you ever have intercourse without coming?
   (Probes: How often? With all partners? Is there any kind of situation that makes it worse?)

3. Has this always been true of you? If not, can you think of anything that might have made things change?
   (Probes: Drug use? Traumatic sexual experience? Partner change?)

4. Are there any circumstances when you do ejaculate?
   (Probes: Masturbation? Oral sex? Anal sex? Other partners? Homosexual partners? Sex aids? Fantasies?)

5. How does your partner react when you take a long time to come?

6. Let's go back in time to your early experiences of intercourse. How were things then?
   (Probes: Partners? Situations? Any problems?)

7. Can you remember any sexual experiences with sex that were upsetting or embarrassing to you?
   (Probes: Erectile dysfunction? Unwilling partner? Rape?)

8. Are you on any medications?

9. Have you had any surgery on or near your sex organs?
   (Probes: Penis? Testicles? Bladder? Prostate?)

Dyspareunia

Painful intercourse for men almost always has an organic cause, such as urethral infection urethral scar tissue resulting from gonorrhoea or a tight foreskin. These can usually be treated directly.

References

1. Channon, L.D, and Ballinger, S.E. Some aspects of sexuality and vaginal symptoms during menopause and their relation to anxiety and depression. *British Journal of Medical Psychology*, 1986: 59, 173–180.
2. Loulan, J. *Lesbian sex*. San Francisco: Spinsters/Aunt Lute, 1984.
3. Comfort, A. *The joy of sex. A gourmet guide*. Mitchell Beazley: London 1987.
4. Bancroft, J and Coles, L. Three years' experience in a sexual problems clinic. *Br Med J*, 1976: 1575–1577.
5. Meares, E. An assessment of the work of 26 doctors trained by the Institute of Psychosexual Medicine. *Public Health*, 1978: 92, 218–223.
6. Masters, W.H, and Johnson, V.E. *Human sexual inadequacy*. Boston: Little, Brown and Co., 1970.
7. Kinsey, A.C, Pomeroy, W.B, Martin, C.E, and Gebhard, P.H. *Sexual behaviour in the human female*. Philadelphia: W.B. Saunders, 1953.

CHAPTER 4

SEXUAL HISTORY TAKING FOR SEXUALLY TRANSMISSIBLE DISEASES

Sexually transmissible diseases (STDs) have, with the publicity in the past decade given to herpes and AIDS, become more familiar to the general population. Despite this, there are still a number of myths about them and the practitioner may need to provide education as much as diagnosis. In particular, many people do not understand that infection may (and commonly does) occur without signs or symptoms. There are also occasionally people who believe that notification of diseases involves public exposure as a punishment for sexual behaviour. For this reason, it is probably more important in taking a history for STDs than for any other area of sexuality to explain the reasons for particular questions. Generally the patient with a suspected STD presents with some suspicion of what the problem may be. On the other hand, there are a number of genital infections which are not, or not necessarily, sexually transmitted. A word on terminology is important here. Sexually transmissible diseases can be transmitted by sexual contact, but also by other means (for example, herpes, syphilis, HIV). Sexually transmitted diseases are usually invariably transmitted by sexual contact (for example, gonorrhoea, genital warts). The distinction is important in both taking a history and explaining to the patient the need for the history or the possible source of infection.

Commencing the history

It is important to put the patient at ease, and this should be done as much as possible while taking the demographic details and history of signs and symptoms. At the same time, a thorough history of recent medication, particularly antibiotics, should also be taken. This is for two reasons: first, because antibiotics may mask the symptoms of any infection, and second, because fixed drug reactions or other effects of medications may mimic the signs of STD infections.

Previous STDs

A history of previous STD infections needs to be taken, and if previous STDs have occurred, it needs to be clear whether these were self-diagnosed and treated, whether a presumptive diagnosis and treatment was made by a health practitioner, or whether the diagnosis was made by laboratory evidence. While this may seem self-evident, it is not uncommon to find that STDs were not definitively diagnosed, and thus the degree of confidence one can have in previous diagnoses is lower. If treatment occurred, it is also useful to determine whether the full course of treatment was followed.

Confidentiality and the law

In many jurisdictions, STDs must be notified to the government health authorities. This is for two reasons. First, this is necessary for epidemiological purposes to attempt to assess the incidence of STD infections and their trend over time. Second, the government may need such information to determine the effectiveness of contact tracing or partner notification.

The purpose of notification, as has already been mentioned, is frequently misunderstood by patients, who do not understand the purposes of epidemiology and fear exposure. We find it is most useful to actually show patients the notification forms if they are in any doubt, and assure them that this information is completely confidential and will only be seen by the health practitioner and by the epidemiologist in the government health department.

A further major concern, particularly where the practice is in a small community, is confidentiality. There have been sufficient situations with HIV infection, particularly in the early days of the epidemic, where infected people have been exposed either in the media or through gossip, with highly distressing and discriminatory results. Absolute confidentiality must be assured and provided, and this fact must be made clear to **all** those working in a practice or clinic, regardless of their role. It only takes one case of breach of confidentiality to ruin one's own reputation and the reputation of one's clinic or practice, and is in addition unethical and could lead to professional censure or withdrawal of a license to practice. These issues are discussed further in the chapter on legal and ethical aspects.

How far back does one take a history?

The short answer to this question is that one takes a history back to the point where the history becomes too uncertain to be reliable. This may vary from a total history for the individual with few sex contacts to a history of the past week for a worker in the sex industry or a prostitute. A second criterion is to consider the incubation period of the disease which is suspected, and to take the longest possible incubation period plus a week. This has, however, a number of limitations.

The major limitation is that where a person is at risk for one STD, they will be at risk for others. It is a well established fact that a significant proportion of patients presenting with STDs may have multiple infections, some of which may be sub-clinical. If an STD if found or suspected, it is important to check for other STDs at the same time.

A further limitation is that because many STDs will be sub-clinical, or 'silent' infections, there is no certainty when the infection occurred. Further, the infection may be clinically intermittent, such as genital herpes. Thus, the patient may have been infected and been infecting other people for a long time. Even with clinical signs of STD infection, infection may have occurred some time previously and have become clinically obvious only because of illness, alteration in immune function, or stress.

A third problem is that some infections, such as HIV or herpes, may have a long incubation time (in the case of HIV, over ten years) and thus it is difficult in some cases to take a full history over this time period, particularly where the person has had a number of sexual partners. A clinical judgement needs to be made in each case as to what will provide the best history with regard to notifying contacts and determining what tests to carry out and where.

History of numbers of sexual partners

The easiest way to take a history of numbers of sexual partners is to obtain estimates first of lifetime sexual partners, then of partners over the past year, and then if this is still a considerable number, of those within the maximum incubation period of the suspected STD (if one or more are suspected).

Once this has been done, the history of partners should be taken backwards, with the most recent first. We find it is helpful to ask the first names only of the partners (if known) or other details to identify them, and their gender.

The issue of partner gender is one where most STD histories founder. It is easy to assume that for a female partners will be a male, and for a male that the partner will be a female. Where one makes this mistake (by asking, for example, 'How many men have you had sex with...' or 'What was his first name?'), one precludes taking a history of homosexual or bisexual sex. This is probably the single most common mistake to occur in taking a sexual history in the context of STDs. Ross[1] found that between 20% and 53% of men with homosexual contacts did not admit to this fact in STD clinics (with more not admitting to such contact in countries where homosexual behaviour was more stigmatised). It is important to make it clear that one is interested in sexual partners of both genders and to explicitly ask, after asking for an estimate of numbers of previous partners, whether these partners were men, women, or both genders.

History of sexual practices

Once the numbers of sexual partners has been established, it is useful to write down the first name or initial of each partner and then go back and fill in the details of the sexual encounter. Because the details of sexual practices are necessary to make an assessment of what sites to investigate for infection, one should first ask what sexual contacts occurred (this should include contacts without ejaculation). Then for each contact, it should be established whether the following sexual activities occurred.

Vaginal intercourse
Was there vaginal penetration by penis, by fingers, or by sex toys such as vibrators or other objects? This latter point is important to assess if vaginal trauma exists or may have occurred. If vaginal sex occurred, vaginal investigations should occur.

Anal intercourse
Was there anal penetration (this must be asked of both male and female patients)? While anal intercourse may occur in homosexual contacts, it is important to note that it has been reported as a sexual practice in 10-20% of heterosexual women and appears to be more common than most practitioners think. If there is any suggestion of anal intercourse, then anal investigation should occur.

Oral sex

Oral sex is probably one of the most common practices in homosexual intercourse,[2] and is also common in heterosexual encounters. It is necessary to establish, first, if oral sex occurred, and second, if it did, who inserted what into whom. The most common practices are likely to be oro-penile sex (fellatio) and oro-vulval sex (cunnilingus). However, oro-anal sex is becoming more common in heterosexual contacts (and should be routinely asked about in cases of homosexual contacts).

Where oro-penile sex has occurred, the urethra and pharynx would be considered for culture. Where oro-vulval and oro-anal sex has occurred, urethral and vaginal and urethral and anal sites should be investigated respectively.

Manual sex and non-penetrative practices

Manual sex is common and may for some people be the preferred form of sexual release. Mutual or non-shared masturbation does not in general pose a risk of STD infection. Nor does frottage (where full body contact may be used to achieve stimulation or orgasm).

Other penetrative practices

These are relatively rare and include the use of sex toys, which may possibly transmit pathogens, and brachioproctic practices. This latter practice may occur in both homosexual and heterosexual contacts, although it has been rarely reported between men and women. While provided there are no tears in the epithelia it is difficult to transmit STDs this way, HIV transmission through brachioproctic sex has been reported by Donovan and colleagues.[3] These practices are reported for the sake of completeness but it is recognised that they will figure in the more specialised practices and not form part of the sexual history in the usual course of events.

Where penetrative practices may lead to trauma, STD transmission may be enhanced and if trauma is suspected, it should be investigated during the physical investigation.

It is important not to make assumptions about the gender of a patient's sexual partners or about which of the range of sexual practices may have occurred, because patients will often be too embarrassed to admit to, say, bisexual or homosexual contact. A leading question which assumes that all contacts are heterosexual will probably in such cases elicit a substantially false history. On the other hand, some practitioners may be understandably embarrassed about appearing to make assumptions in the other direction. We find it is helpful to preface the history of sexual practices by a comment such as 'I am going to ask you about a range of sexual practices which we commonly have reported to us'. This will usually put the patient more at ease and make it less difficult or embarrassing to report on practices which they may feel ashamed about. We also prefer to refer to **'partner(s)'** (genderless) and only later after the history has commenced ask about the gender if this is still unclear. The patient will almost invariably fill in the gaps by referring to the partner as 'he' or 'she', thus obviating the need for a direct question!

Condom use and contraception

Following on from the history of sexual practices, or at the same time if it is easier, the clinician should ascertain whether condoms were used. It is important not to assume that condom use implies protection. If the condom was put on at the last minute, infection still may have occurred since ejaculation is not a necessary condition for STD infection. Further, inappropriate or inadequate fitting of the condom as well as breakage may also lead to infection. This possibility should be explored.

In some patients, there may be the belief that contraception (particularly douche, spermicide or barrier methods such as the diaphragm) may preclude infection. Alternatively, where an IUD is fitted, particularly those (no longer commonly used) with a filamentous tail, infection of the pelvis should be considered and an appropriate history taken or examination performed.

Compliance

While taking a sexual history, it is also useful to form an opinion as to whether the patient is likely to be compliant with treatment regimens. This can be ascertained through previous histories of compliance with medication or determining whether their social situation is likely to place any barriers in the path of compliance with treatment.

Partner Notification

Partner notification (also known as contact tracing) is frequently a source of concern to the patient and an obligation (in some places a legal one) of the practitioner. However, research has suggested that the most accurate partner notification is done by the patient.[4] If the patient does not want a particular partner to be notified, they will withhold information which will make such notification impossible. At times, there will simply not be enough information available to identify the partner (for example, 'He was about my height and left handed. We met behind the City Tavern').

The patient needs to be given the options, where partners are identifiable, to either make the notification themselves, or to have the practitioner do it for them (anonymously if preferred). In some cases, patients will have real fears of retribution or discrimination where their identity is made known to the contact, and the practitioner should respect such concerns.

In such cases, if the patient chooses not to notify the contact themselves, the practitioner can send out a form letter stating that 'You may have been exposed to an infectious disease through contact with a carrier. Please contact (the clinic or practitioner) quoting the number above so that we can arrange to investigate any possible infections and treat them where appropriate.' Alternatively, many STD clinics have specialised facilities for contact tracing and may be happy to have any contacts referred on to them. This may have the additional advantage of preserving anonymity if it is possible for the contact to identify the patient from the clinic or practitioner they attend.

In general, if patients are willing to have partners notified, it is far more cost-effective to have them do it themselves (cards or letters may be given them for this purpose). If patients are unwilling to have contacts notified, they will simply not cooperate and attempting to force them to do so will simply alienate them and lead to lack of compliance or avoidance of attendance for future screening or symptoms.

Concluding the interview

At the conclusion of the history, it is important to debrief the client from what may have been an embarrassing or difficult interview. This debriefing should commence with a summary (in appropriate language) of what steps are likely to be taken next in terms of investigations or treatment.

Following this, it is also important to give the patient a chance to add anything (we are all familiar with the patient who brings up a major issue in the last minutes of a consultation). Sometimes the patient will want to correct information, or to make an admission that they were not entirely forthcoming once they have ascertained that the practitioner is accepting and does not make moral judgements. Clinicians who work full time in STD practices are familiar with such occasions ('Actually, I did have sex with another man once ...').

The other important purpose of the time for questions at the end of the history is to provide the patient with an opportunity to ask questions which may be able to correct fears or misapprehensions, such as whether their behaviour is 'normal', or what the effects of STDs may be on fertility, or what the signs and symptoms of particular STDS may be. It is important to allow these questions both from the point of debriefing and clarification, and also from the point of leading into preventive education (described in a later chapter).

In summary, the STD history is designed to give the practitioner the information needed to carry out appropriate investigations, make an appropriate diagnosis, and to carry out appropriate partner and epidemiological notification. It can also prepare the groundwork for preventive education. As with all sexual histories, the key to success is to take a non-judgemental attitude, explain to the patient why you are asking particular questions, and be clear why you need to ask particular questions and where they may lead you in terms of their clinical implications. Even if the decision is to refer the patient on, it will be a great help to the practitioner you refer on to have a clear and concise history and possible differential diagnoses to start from.

References

1. Ross, M.W. Psychosocial factors in admitting to homosexuality in sexually transmitted disease clinics. *Sex Transm Dis*, 1985: 12, 83–86.
2. Ross, M.W. *Psychovenereology*. New York: Praeger, 1986.
3. Donovan, B, Tindall, B.D and Cooper, D.A. Brachioproctic eroticism and transmission of the AIDS retrovirus. *Genitourinary Medicine*, 1986: 62, 390–392.
4. Rothenberg, R.B and Potterat, J.J. Strategies for management of sexual partners. In: Holmes, K.K., Mårdh, P.A, Sparling, P.F and Wiesner, P.J. (eds) *Sexually transmitted diseases* (2nd edn). New York: McGraw-Hill, 1990: 1081–1086.

CHAPTER 5

SEXUAL COUNSELLING

Modern counselling is a situation where a therapist and client together explore and delineate the client's problem, set attainable goals for therapy and devise strategies to reach those goals.

Counselling theory and practice has two main sources: the work of Carl Rogers[1,2] and modern learning theory.

Let's begin with Rogers. He believes that human beings have an innate potential for positive personality change. He called it **self-actualisation**. The role of the helping professional is simply to provide the client with a situation where growth can occur.

He saw three essential ingredients that any therapist needs to provide.[3]

- Respect and regard for the client. While we may not always approve of everything the client does or says, we need to convey the fact that we believe he or she is basically a decent human being with the capacity to develop and grow.
- Empathic understanding. This is the willingness to listen carefully to the client, see things from his or her point of view and to communicate the understanding.
- Genuineness (congruence). This is the therapist's feeling of being comfortable with him or herself and being able to respond spontaneously.

The implication of this approach is that the counsellor is a facilitator, who helps the patient to generate his or her own goals and strategies.

Rogers's greatest contribution to counselling is his emphasis on process. When we look at content, especially for sexual counselling, a behavioural approach is seen to be most productive.

The behavioural approach sprang from learning theory and has several characteristics:

- Much of human behaviour is learned.
- Maladaptive behaviour can be unlearned or more positive behaviours substituted.

- Although maladaptive behaviours were learned in the person's past, therapy focuses on the learning of new behaviours in the here and now.

In terms of sexual counselling, that means that we can focus on a specific problem and treat that, rather than become involved in attempts to promote major personality change.

In addition to these two facets of general counselling, the sexual counsellor has a major role as an **educator**. In spite of the vast amounts of sexual information available in books, magazines, school programmes and so on, much of the population remains in what Packard[4] called 'The Sexual Wilderness', surrounded by rapid changes in attitudes and values, myths and misinformation.

This implies that it is a paramount responsibility of the sex counsellor to be well informed. And to be willing to say, 'I don't know but I'll try to find out', when a question outside your knowledge base turns up.

Useful, practical books to enhance your counselling skills include Egan[5] and Nelson-Jones.[6]

Couples therapy

If at all possible, see both members of a partnership together. This may need a little tact to arrange, especially if one member believes it is the other person's problem. Nonetheless, any sexual difficulty will impact on a relationship and a partner's response to problems may play a part in maintaining and increasing the dysfunction.

Some therapies involve a major commitment of the partner to the treatment programme (see chapter six). Here it is essential to see the partner to maintain motivation, defuse problems and monitor progress.

The commonest scenario in sex counselling is that the patient presents alone. When the history has been taken, point out to the patient that you have been asking about the partner's response a lot of the time. The vast majority of sexual problems are experienced as relationship problems. For this reason and the possible involvement of him or her in treatment, you would like to talk to the partner. Reassure the patient that everything that has already been discussed by the two of you will remain confidential (see chapter twelve).

It's a good idea to seek the patient's permission to telephone the partner and arrange an appointment. There are two good reasons for this. Firstly, it puts a degree of medical 'clout' behind the request. A partner is more likely to refuse to attend if the issue is broached by the original patient. Secondly, it goes a way towards defusing the idea that the therapist and the presenting patient are in an alliance against the partner.

Take a sexual history from the partner in an individual session.

When you see the couple together, make it clear that they are to have equal air space. 'I'm going to ask you, X, to describe things as you see them. Then I'll ask you, Y, to tell me how they affect you'.

Even if a partner refuses to attend your rooms, it is unusual to find a person who is unwilling to take part in even a brief telephone interview.

Masters and Johnson[7] predicated their work on a co-therapist setting, with each member of the couple having a same-sex therapist. The logistics of arranging this are often difficult in a general practice setting and it is far from essential, especially in brief counselling.

Therapist skills

The main points of importance are that the therapist be comfortable in the counselling situation and knowledgeable about sexuality. The skills of active listening, rapport-building and accurate empathy are central, too.

Some of these skills are common to all counselling situations, some more specific to sexual counselling.

Comfort

It is very unproductive for a practitioner to be obviously uncomfortable and evasive when discussing sexual matters. Even if you personally would prefer not to include sexuality in your work with patients, you will undoubtedly find situations where the patients themselves raise sexual matters.

Box 5A gives an example of a practitioner who was evasive in the face of a relatively simple question from a patient.

It's a good idea to desensitise yourself to any embarrassment you feel by doing practice interviews and role plays with colleagues and friends.

Knowledge

As we have said before, it is the responsibility of the practitioner to know as much as possible about the area. Most medical libraries have several texts on sexual problems (many shelved at Dewey number 616.8583).

> **BOX 5A**
>
> ### An uncomfortable practitioner
>
> After repeated dilation and curettage had failed to reduce excessive menstrual bleeding, her gynaecologist recommended that Mrs. C. have a hysterectomy. She went home, discussed the matter with her husband and returned with a series of questions. One of these was, 'Will sex still be as good with me on top?'
>
> She described the gynaecologist's response. 'He nearly fell off his chair, muttered that he didn't know and started asking a heap of questions about other things. He might at least have offered to try and find out.'

Papers on sexual matters can be found in journals of psychiatry, psychology, gynaecology, urology and general medicine. *The Archives of Sexual Behaviour, Journal of Sex and Marital Therapy* and *Medical Aspects of Human Sexuality* are among several specialised journals.

There are innumerable sex manuals in the popular press. Read as much as possible.

Rapport-building

The client needs to feel comfortable before he or she will feel able to discuss sexual matters frankly. The major ingredient here is a calm, professional approach. Feeling comfortable about your own sexuality and that of others is essential.

The physical set-up of your rooms can facilitate communication. For sexual interviews, it's a good idea to seat yourself and the patient in similar sized chairs set at right angles. This reduces formality, is less confrontational and allows the patient to avoid eye contact with you from time to time if he or she wishes.

Two essential ingredients of rapport-building are active listening and accurate empathy.

Active listening

You can communicate the fact that you are listening carefully and actively trying to understand what you hear by both non-verbal and verbal means.

Body language is very important in conveying that we are attending closely to what a person is saying. Egan[5] suggests five behaviours which you can adopt to signify a listening attitude (see Box 5B).

BOX 5B

Non-verbal indicators of listening

- Face the client squarely. (We do not agree with this.) Perhaps it is more acceptable in a North American context.
- Adopt an open posture. Crossed legs and arms signal that you are defensive.
- Lean towards the client.
- Maintain good eye contact. This does not mean that you should stare at the client, but it does suggest that you look at the client when he or she is talking.
- Try to relax.

The verbal behaviours which indicate active listening include such things as the occasional 'yes' or 'um', prompting the patient to continue talking. Do not be too afraid of silences. If you lean toward the patient and look expectant, the chances are that the story will continue. Silence is one of the most potent open-ended questions in your repertoire.

Encourage clients to be specific about issues. This helps them know what you want to hear. If a patient has described an erectile failure experience, you can encourage detail and specificity by a question like, 'I know you felt tense when you got into bed with Sue and couldn't get an erection. Was there something about the situation that started you off feeling that way?'

Reflecting back what the client has said is also helpful. First, it shows that you have been listening. Secondly, it acts as a check that you have understood what has been said. A patient describes inhibitions resulting from parents-in-law being in the next bedroom. 'Right, so you feel uncomfortable that they might hear you, huh?'

Accurate empathy

Empathy is the ability to see the world from the client's perspective. This implies an understanding of what the client has experienced and how he or she reacted emotionally. Not only do you need to be able to see the world from the client's point of view, but you need to communicate your understanding.

Again, summarising and reflecting back are excellent ways of communicating your willingness to see things from the client's point of view.

References

1. Rogers, C.R. *Client-centered therapy*. Boston: Houghton Mifflin, 1951.
2. Rogers, C.R. *On becoming a person*. Boston: Houghton Mifflin, 1961.
3. Rogers, C.R. The necessary and sufficient conditions of therapeutic personality change. *Journal of Consulting Psychology*, 1957: 21, 95–104.
4. Packard, V. *The sexual wilderness*. London: Longmans, Green and Company, 1968.
5. Egan, G. *The skilled helper. Models, skills and methods of effective helping*. (2nd edn). Monterey: Brooks/Cole, 1982.
6. Nelson-Jones, R. *Theory and practice of counselling psychology*. Eastbourne: Holt, Rinehart and Winston, 1982.
7. Masters, W.H and Johnson, V.E. *Human sexual inadequacy*. Boston: Little, Brown and Company, 1970.

CHAPTER 6

SEXUAL COUNSELLING AND TREATMENT

This chapter outlines the PLISSIT model of sexual counselling.[1] It also suggests interventions for some of the more commonly encountered dysfunctions.

The PLISSIT model

The PLISSIT model suggests that interventions in sexual dysfunctions can occur at four levels of complexity.

Box 6A outlines the levels of intervention.

BOX 6A

The PLISSIT model

- **P**ermission to talk about sexual matters, fantasise, enjoy sexuality.
- **L** imited
  I nformation
- **S** pecific
  S uggestions
- **I** ntensive
  T herapy

Annon and Robinson, 1978

Permission: At this level the practitioner introduces questions about the patient's sexuality (or, more rarely, responds to sexual questions or information volunteered by the patient). These actions establish that it is totally appropriate to discuss sexual matters in a medical setting, that the practitioner is able and willing to clarify the issues involved and to initiate treatment if necessary.

Limited information: may be all that is needed. We have found that the most valuable limited information is a short account of differences in the typical male and female sexual response:

- Women take longer to warm up sexually. There is a need for protracted foreplay, starting with non-genital contact.
- Women also take longer to cool down. Rolling over and going to sleep immediately after ejaculation is simply not good enough.
- Men find direct genital stimulation pleasurable and arousing even before they have attained an erection.
- Women find direct stimulation of the clitoris highly unpleasant if they have not reached a state of sexual arousal. Ouch.

Another important area of limited information concerns the possible effects of medication on erectile functioning. Physicians are sometimes reluctant to warn male patients that a drug may reduce erectile capacity. They believe that a man may expect failure, become anxious and thus ensure an erectile disaster. We think it better to explain that in some cases the drug may affect erection. You can tell the patient that if it does, there is a possibility of substituting another drug or lowering the dosage. This increases the probability that the patient will report back if he is having problems rather than just accepting the situation or taking himself off the medication.

Specific suggestions: Some of them, like sensate focus exercises, can be used in a wide variety of situations. Others, like the squeeze technique in premature ejaculation, have a more specialised application. These suggestions are discussed below.

Intensive therapy: is usually provided by a specialist sex therapist. It is indicated when there is major accompanying psychopathology, substance abuse, major relationship discord or in any case when the primary physician feels out of his or her depth.

Referral

There are two opposing considerations to be weighed in the balance when you are considering referring a patient to a specialist sex therapist. Certainly, the patient may receive more sophisticated and perhaps longer term treatment. On the other hand, it is easy for the patient to perceive referral as rejection. Especially for the patient who has had difficulties and doubts about mentioning sexual matters, it may seem as if he or she has overstepped the mark of acceptability. The referral may also be seen as confirmation that the patient has something pretty drastically wrong.

Treating sexual dysfunctions

Sensate focus exercises

These can be employed in a wide variety of situations with flexible use of the rules. They can be used to enhance sexual enjoyment in a situation where no dysfunction exists, in orgasmic dysfunction, premature and retarded ejaculation and so on. Box 6B gives a summary of the exercises, but a fuller account is given by Masters and Johnson[2] and Kaplan.[3]

BOX 6B

Sensate focus exercises

The couple lie together naked on a comfortable surface where they can ensure privacy (even if it means fitting a bolt to the door). One partner lies on his or her stomach while the other systematically strokes him or her from the back of the head to the toes, taking time over each body part. The role of the stroker is to experiment with different kinds of touching, that of the receiver to focus on enjoyment of body responses and to give a little feedback about what he or she finds pleasurable.

When either partner chooses, the receiver turns over and the partner begins sensual fondling of the front of the body, avoiding the breasts and genitals. (Most authorities confine themselves to suggesting avoiding a female's breasts, but male nipples can be highly charged erogenous zones too.)

When either partner decides, the roles are reversed.

The rules at this stage are simple:

- No genital or nipple touching.
- No intercourse.
- Tell your partner what you like (and what you don't).
- Don't rush.

The partners are asked to carry out the exercise two or three times before their next appointment with the practitioner.

When both partners are ready, they may include nipple and genital touching, but the rule about no intercourse continues.

It may happen in either of the two first stages that one or both partners becomes sexually aroused. If so, they should masturbate afterwards, alone if that can be arranged.

Again, when both partners are good and ready, they can progress to intercourse, but without any pressure to reach orgasm.

Derived from Masters and Johnson (1970)

The exercises have many uses:

- To enable people to get to know their own and their partner's preferred placing, timing and kind of tactile stimulation.
- To enable sexually-anxious people to relax with each other.
- To reduce pressure to perform.
- As part of a planned dysfunction treatment programme.

The exercises are 'homework'. Couples are asked to try them out two or three times between sessions. They then discuss their responses to the exercises in the therapy period.

The couple move gradually through the exercises at their own pace. In the beginning, stimulation of genitals and breasts is off-limits. When the two are comfortable with this level, they move along to genital touching but with intercourse still prohibited.

The therapist and couple together decide the level at which they can comfortably start. Very sexually anxious people are encouraged to begin by lying down fully-clothed and kissing and cuddling.

We see no reason not to use massage oil in these exercises. There are many varieties of oil on the market, or cold-pressed almond oil with a dash of scented herb oil is also good. **NEVER** introduce oil-based products into the vagina.

An important component of the exercises is to discourage what Masters and Johnson[2] call 'spectatoring'. That is the anxious monitoring of one's sexual functioning, worries about how the partner is responding and so on.

In the next section we look at specific sexual dysfunctions and approaches to treatment.

Erectile dysfunction

Having decided that the causes of erectile dysfunction are not organic (see chapter three) you need to determine what psychological factors are, or have been, operating. We say, 'or have been' because it not infrequently happens that a single episode of erectile failure produces anxiety at the next attempt. This reduces the chance of a functional erection and a vicious cycle is set up.

All kinds of things can trigger off a failure experience. One patient described the super-tidy flat of his mistress-to-be. 'Even her jumpers were all folded up in those little basket things. I just couldn't get it up'.

Common factors include the particular partner, the situation and the patient's attitudes (see Box 6C).

BOX 6C

Triggers for erectile failure

Features of the partner

- A partner of the non-preferred sex.
- A physically unattractive partner (obesity, ageing, not good looking, inverted nipples, etc.)
- A moody, cross, irritable, tense or preoccupied partner
- A poor relationship
- A passive, unenthusiastic or unwilling partner

Features of the situation

- Lack of privacy, possibility of interruption
- Guilt about infidelity
- Desire to impress a new partner
- Overuse of drugs or alcohol
- Medication effects
- Alertness for crying children

Features of the man

- Anxiety about previous failures
- Spectatoring tendency

When a psychological cause or causes is found, it should be directly treated. The **permission** level of the PLISSIT model is important as the practitioner encourages the patient to tease out the components that led to erectile failure in the first place. **Limited information** about the feedback loop where anxiety leads to a greater chance of failure and the role of spectatoring is also helpful.

The role of the counsellor is to help the patient identify the factors which triggered off the original failure experience. If those components are still present, what can be done? A sexually-passive partner may be encouraged to take a more active role. Bolts can be fitted to bedroom doors. The occasional visit to a motel can be undertaken. All sorts of minor, practical adjustments can be made.

Perhaps the most salient intervention is to initiate **sensate focus exercises** with a co-operative and attractive partner. When the man finds that he can enjoy sensual experiences with no pressure to proceed to intercourse, there is a good chance that he will begin to have erections again. If his partner is female, the woman on top position is possibly the easiest way to restart intercourse. It does not necessarily require a full erection and is easier to incorporate into sensate focus exercises.

Surgical prophylaxes: In cases of organically-based dysfunction or psychogenic dysfunction which does not respond to treatment (relatively rare), surgical implants may be considered. This usually necessitates referral to a urological surgeon.

Premature ejaculation

As we said earlier (see chapter three), it is difficult to define premature ejaculation. Usually, the best operational definition is the fact that the patient and his partner complain about it. (Though there is the story of the patient who was asked to be more specific about his problem. 'After quarter of an hour or so, I just can't stop it'.)

Many men take their own initiatives to delay ejaculation. Box 6D gives a rather disastrous example of this approach. It also illustrates the need for communication between sexual partners.

BOX 6D

A failure of communication

Mr. D.'s preferred technique for delaying orgasm was to recite the teams of the English Football League to himself, beginning with the fourth division. He would utter early warning signals from time to time. ('I'm up to Charlton Athletic, love'.) He would eventually collapse, with a triumphant cry of, 'Liverpool!'.

He and his wife, who was orgasmically dysfunctional, had seemingly never discussed this behaviour. Mr. D. was upset about the dysfunction and rather angry considering his heroic efforts.

In a conjoint session, Mrs. D. volunteered that she would prefer him to come at any time he chose, as she didn't find intercourse stimulating anyway. During intercourse she tended to plan meals and marketing for the following week.

Therapy focussed on sexual enjoyment and increased foreplay, with Mrs. D. reaching orgasm before intercourse started.

There are two major categories of treatment. One, aimed at increased ejaculatory control, can be described as the 'P.E.'s a disease' approach. The other is designed to allow the couple to enjoy their sexual experiences without focussing on ejaculation.

While many couples want to prolong intercourse, the second approach is quicker, easier and relatively fail-safe.

The usual approaches to enhancing ejaculatory control involve some combination of three techniques:

- Graded sensate focus exercises.
- Semans'[14] technique.
- Masters and Johnsons'[2] squeeze technique.

The initial step, as always, is **permission**. The partners need permission to talk about their experiences. They also need permission to enjoy sensuality and sexuality, especially where one or both have guilt feelings about sex.

Limited information can include the fact that most men ejaculate within two minutes of intromission.[4] The patient can be reassured, however, that if he and his partner are willing to cooperate, he can learn to delay ejaculation. At this point the patient's early experience of situations where it was important to come quickly (furtive masturbation, danger of invasion of privacy, use of workers in the sex industry for whom time is money, etc.) may be valuable as a justification of the re-learning approach.

Specific suggestions : Initially, a graded set of sensate focus exercises combined with Semans' technique can be outlined (see Box 6E). The couple should try to do the exercises at least twice in the week before the next appointment.

We need to say a word about sexual satisfaction of both partners in the early stages of the programme. It is better, if it is acceptable to them, that they masturbate in private after finishing the exercises if they feel the need.

Certainly, the programme is very demanding, especially for the partner. You need to be completely honest about this before they begin, as failure experiences can be demoralising and destructive.

You also need to tell the couple that in the early stages of the programme, when the man is less in tune with the sensations leading up to ejaculation he may accidentally come. If this happens, they simply suspend operations for a while.

BOX 6E

Semans' technique and sensate focus exercises

The couple lie naked together and the patient's partner touches his body, avoiding the genital and nipples, until he gets an erection. The partner continues stimulation until the man signals that he is close to ejaculation. The partner then ceases stimulation until the ejaculatory urge (and perhaps the erection) subsides. The partner then begins again and repeats the procedure two or three times.

The instructions given to the man are that he should be totally and utterly selfish. He focuses on his own sensual and sexual responses and on telling his partner when he begins to feel the ejaculatory urge.

Once the couple can manage this step satisfactorily, they move on to a similar procedure that now involves genital and nipple stimulation. Again, the partner ceases stimulation when the man signals the ejaculatory urge.

In later sessions, when the patient gains a firm erection, he inserts it into his partner, but does not make any pelvic movements. At the ejaculatory urge, he withdraws and lies quietly until the urge subsides. This is repeated two or three times.

The next step is to incorporate slight pelvic thrusting, but again to withdraw at the start of the ejaculatory urge.

Rationale

This programme is rather similar to Wolpe and Lazarus's[15] systematic desensitisation technique for the treatment of phobias. There, progressively stronger phobic stimuli are introduced when the patient is in a state incompatible with anxiety, such as relaxation.

The programme allows the man to become more aware of his sexual responses, especially those relating to ejaculation, and gradually deconditions the early ejaculation behaviour.

The Masters and Johnson[2] squeeze technique can be used as a quick means of suppressing the ejaculatory urge. (For some reason most books illustrate this by a hand with dangerously long fingernails.) When the patient feels the ejaculatory urge, his partner grasps his penis firmly, thumb on the frenulum, first two fingers on the head of the penis, and squeezes. It's a good idea for the patient to give feedback about the amount of pressure to be used. Most partners are initially reluctant to squeeze hard enough. Warn the couple that the patient's erection will probably subside to a degree.

We might add that the success rate for fully cooperative couples is almost a hundred percent.

Other approaches: It seems to us that Australian couples are less willing than their North American counterparts to engage in the sexual heroics of a sensate focus programme.

Anyway, contrary to popular belief, many female partners do not particularly enjoy having a man bounce up and down on them for extended periods of time. This is especially true for a woman who tends not to be orgasmic with intercourse (see Box 6D).

For these couples, therapy can focus on enhancing enjoyment of sexual relations without the rigorous re-learning of ejaculatory control.

There are several **specific suggestions** which can enhance a couple's sexual enjoyment. Give them a choice.

- Buy a good guide to sex. For heterosexuals, nothing in our opinion has outshone Comfort's *Joy of Sex*.[5] Silverstein and White's *Joy of Gay Sex*[6] is a good manual for gay men.
- Make sure the partner comes, by manual, oral or any other congenial form of stimulation before the patient inserts his penis.
- Have the patient stimulate his partner almost to orgasm, insert his penis, lie still and continue to stimulate the partner.
- Have the patient ejaculate quickly once. Wait a while (a few minutes with younger men, an hour or so with older men) and make love again with lots of foreplay. This makes use of what Masters and Johnson call the relative refractory period — a time when a man is able to reach orgasm but slower in doing so.
- Use condoms, especially ones with ribs and 'ticklers'. The reduced sensation can often delay male orgasm.
- Play sensate focus games with relaxed rules.

Retarded ejaculation

Much retarded ejaculation results from medication side effects. As we said, it is really only fair to warn the patient of this possibility when the drug is prescribed. This warning is the equivalent of **permission** to discuss any sexual problems that may arise from using the drug. If problems do arise, the need is to balance therapeutic gains against side effects, with due reference to the needs of the patient. A related drug may not affect ejaculation. A lower dosage may be sufficient for clinical gains.

Medications (notably some anti-psychotics) may also produce dry ejaculation. Semen enters the bladder rather than the urethra. The same balancing of priorities and considerations of alternatives apply.

With organically-caused retarded ejaculation there may simply be no solution other than surgery. That does not imply that you give up on the patient. Counselling of a supportive nature and **specific suggestions** about sexual activities that do not necessarily involve male orgasm are important.

Generally we would recommend that retarded ejaculators whose problem is psychogenic be referred to a specialist sex therapist. The complex interaction of sexual, emotional and situational factors takes more time to analyse and work through than is available in most general practice situations.

If referral is not an option, say in a remote country practice, we suggest that you find out when the man can ejaculate, if at all. If he is completely unable to ejaculate in the presence of a partner, make every effort to refer him to a specialist therapist. If he is able to masturbate to orgasm in the presence of a partner, this can form part of sensate focus exercises. Eventually the partner's hand is placed over the patient's hand as he masturbates. The couple progess to masturbation with the partner's hand alone. This requires willingness on the part of the patient to communicate what he needs at any given time.

Men's masturbation procedures vary remarkably from person to person and at different stages in the response cycle. A man may start out needing long, slow strokes from the shaft to the head, modified to the shaft only as the head becomes more sensitive, culminating in fast stimulation of the whole penis as ejaculation nears. How is a partner to guess?

Once masturbation by the partner is achieved, the couple can proceed through the sensate focus exercises to intercourse if they wish.

Female organic dysfunction (anorgasmia and generalised orgasmic dysfunction)

The first need is to check whether the woman is only non-orgasmic during intercourse or whether she has orgasms during other activities such as masturbation, manual or oral stimulation or erotic dreams. If concurrent orgasmic capacity is established, the way ahead is much easier.

The **limited information** to be passed on is that perhaps the majority of women do not reach orgasm during intercourse unless there is some direct stimulation of the clitoris, say by her or her partner's hand.

As with premature ejaculation, one possibility is for the couple to accept that she is not going to reach orgasm easily in the intercourse situation. The couple can focus on plenty of foreplay, moving up to manual and oral stimulation of the clitoris, so that the woman reaches orgasm before intercourse begins.

If the couple are determined that they want the woman to reach orgasm in an intercourse situation, **specific suggestions** can be made. The couple can embark on graded sensate focus exercises and, if both partners agree, the woman can start masturbation practice.

You can tell the couple that female orgasm is caused by is stimulation of the clitoris, an organ very like a small penis. It is important that the woman be aroused sexually by non-genital touching, kissing and cuddling before her partner touches her clitoris. It is downright unpleasant to be touched directly on an unaroused clitoris.

While clitoral stimulation is the direct cause of orgasm, there are many possible inhibitors. Some of them are listed in Box 6F.

You might point out that masturbation is perfectly normal. The Kinsey Report on female sexuality[7] found that over half of their sample masturbated. With the relaxing of attitudes to sex in the last thirty five years, one might expect that a higher proportion of women today are prepared to admit that they masturbate.

Masturbation may also be a positive health benefit. The increased flow of blood to the genitals in masturbation and intercourse helps maintain the vaginal epithelium, especially in post-menopausal women. It may also enhance orgasmic capacity.

You should also point out that the myth of a distinction between vaginal and clitoral orgasms is just that — a myth.

You need to give the woman **permission** to use sexual aids such as books and magazines. Comfort's *Joy of Sex*[5] is a sensible, warmly-written guide. Loulan's books, *Lesbian Sex*[8] and *Lesbian Passion*[9] are useful for homosexual and bisexual women. (Not that heterosexuals cannot learn a lot from them too.) Fantasies are also helpful. Fantasies such as semi-public lovemaking (surreptitious stimulation under the tablecloth at a dinner party, for example), making love outdoors, and so on, are common female fantasies that can increase arousal.

An electric vibrator may be a help at first, though the woman will need to progress to manual stimulation eventually.

The woman should masturbate two or three times a week in a situation where she is comfortable. She needs to focus on what kinds of body stimulation are pleasurable to her. Especially when women

> **BOX 6F**
>
> ## Factors inhibiting female orgasm
>
> *Features of the patient*
>
> - Guilt about sex
> - Anxiety and tension
> - Anger and hostility
> - Depression
> - Tiredness
> - Spectatoring
> - Concerns about possible pregnancy
> - Pelvic pain
>
> *Features of the situation*
>
> - Possibility of interruption
> - Guilt about infidelity
> - Alertness for crying children
> - Physical discomfort (eg a small parked car)
> - Distractions (eg noisy neighbours)
> - Marital discord
> - Reluctance to have intercourse
>
> *Features of the partner*
>
> - Physically unattractive
> - Poor sexual technique
> - Sexual dysfunction
> - Preferences for distasteful or uncomfortable acts
> - Not the preferred sex

have breast fed children, concurrent stimulation of a nipple and the clitoris may be exquisitely pleasurable. She should avoid spectatoring and the feeling that she **must** reach orgasm every time she masturbates. A water-soluble lubricant such as K-Y Jelly may be useful in avoiding soreness.

When she is comfortable with masturbation, aware of what kinds of touching suits her and able to reach orgasm on at least some of the occasions, genital fondling may be incorporated into the sensate focus exercises if she chooses and her partner agrees. She should guide her partner about what pleases her, where she wants to be touched and how. She can demonstrate what kind of touching works best. (Many men are sexually aroused by the sight of a woman masturbating.)

The next step is to initiate orgasm with the man's penis in the woman's vagina. As the woman nears orgasm she should stimulate the partner's penis to erection. She then straddles him as he continues to stimulate her and inserts his penis just as she reaches orgasm.

The length of time of penis insertion can be gradually increased, still using the woman-on-top position, as this makes it easier for the man to continue direct clitoral stimulation when the penis is inserted.

For women who have never masturbated to orgasm, the programme should start at a much gentler level. A non-threatening beginning to learning about body responses is to focus on them in the shower. Encourage the woman to use a good shower gel or exfoliating cream. She gets wet, turns off the shower and then smoothes the cream over her body, paying attention to the sensuality of the experience and her bodily sensations. To repeat, creams, oils and lotions should **NEVER** be put in the vagina.

One of the authors (LDC-L) finds that a productive, **permission**-giving approach is to use imagery in hypnosis. The woman is encouraged to imagine the scene as vividly as possible, 'almost as if you were really there'. Non-sexual images should be evoked, for example the luxury of sitting up in bed on a sunny morning and stretching every muscle, feeling the warm sun and the texture of the sand as she lies on a beach, or the shower scene. The woman is encouraged to enjoy and be pleased with the feelings her body can produce.

She can then move on at her own pace to genital touching without the aim of orgasm and then to the programme described above.

As with most aspects of lesbian women's health, there is little hard data on orgasmic dysfunction. Even if epidemiological data were available, one would have to question its validity. We suspect that lesbian women would be relatively reluctant to present with sexual problems to a predominantly heterosexual and still rather male dominated profession.

It was our gut-feeling that lesbian couples may have less orgasmic dysfunction than heterosexual couples. Our reasons for this are:

- So much limited information which proves to be therapeutic in counselling heterosexual couples is straight forward education about differences between men and women in terms of sexual response

cycles. A woman can apply her knowledge of her own responses to the likely feelings of her partner.
- Perhaps a woman would be more understanding of the fact that a female partner can enjoy sex without reaching orgasm. A fair proportion of women who are not orgasmic present on the insistence of their male partners who feel that they, the men, are failures if the woman does not reach orgasm.
- Oral and manual stimulation, major components in lesbian sexuality, are far more likely to lead to orgasm than is a short period of foreplay followed by intercourse.

On the other hand, Loulan,[8] a lesbian sex therapist, describes orgasmic difficulties in her patients. They include:

- Anorgasmia.
- Orgasm by masturbation, but not with a partner.
- Differing response speed of the partners.

Loulan suggests masturbation practice and a variety of sensate focus style exercises. She also suggests that women remove themselves from what she calls the tyranny of orgasm as a goal in love making. 'Orgasm is highly overrated'. This attitude of mind seems an excellent way to remove performance pressure and might well be incorporated into heterosexual therapy.

We suggest that you read Loulan's books[8,9] before treating a lesbian patient. You can also refer her to the homework exercises towards the end of the earlier book.

Vaginismus

Vaginismus is best treated by referral to a specialist sex therapist. Of course, this is not always possible.

The approach to vaginismus involves three aspects:

- Relaxation techniques.
- Permission to enjoy sexuality and encouragement of this.
- The insertion of progressively larger objects into the vagina.

We find that teaching the woman to relax, with or without hypnosis, is a useful beginning. The imagery suggested above for non-orgasmic women is appropriate.

Goldberg[10] suggests a structured programme. The practitioner explains the rationale of the treatment using the analogy of lift phobia.

It is essential to stress that the patient will be moving along at her own pace and will not be rushed.

Therapy will aim at change in three areas:

- Removing the physical spasm of the muscles.
- The woman's feelings of anxiety or resentment about penetration.
- The woman's concerns that she is abnormal.

As homework, the woman listens to a hypnosis or relaxation tape in the morning. The tape contains sensual imagery of the kind we have described plus desensitising imagery.

In the evening, she listens to a similar tape while in the bath. When the tape has finished, she begins on a series of graded finger penetration exercises, starting with the little finger inserted one knuckle at a time. There is no pressure for achievement. 'The programme is given by the therapist, the pace decided by the client'.

Sessions with the couple together commence as soon as the woman begins to make some progress. Counselling focuses on the fact that both partners are concerned about the painful effects of penetration. 'Otherwise you might be here complaining of rape, not vaginismus'.

Some authorities (e.g. Murjack and Oziel[11]) suggest that the practitioner should demonstrate the insertion of a lubricated finger into the woman's vagina and then the insertion of the smallest of a series of graded dilators. The partner is invited to watch the procedure.

The advantage of this approach is that the woman leaves the doctor's rooms with a success experience. The disadvantage may be that it further lowers the self-esteem of her partner. He has been trying to achieve penetration for some time and may perceive the practitioner's success as belittling. It can also be perceived as a very sexually-charged doctor¢patient situation.

We believe that, on balance, it is better to allow the woman to carry out the whole insertion progress. The notion that the client is responsible for change as far as possible is one of the fundamentals of modern counselling.

Infertility

Of course, infertility cannot be regarded as a sexual dysfunction as such except in special cases, such as the situation where the man suffers retarded ejaculation and fakes orgasm. It is, however, an important area and one where patients need a great deal of support. This is especially

BOX 6G

Infertility: a case history

In early 1975, Mr. and Mrs. R decided to have a family. They had been happily married for three years. He was aged 30 and she 31. She discontinued taking her (high dosage) contraceptive pill and began to take her waking temperature. The couple took care to have intercourse several times when she noted a mid-cycle temperature rise. Her cycle varied between 26 and 40 days.

After a year of trying, they consulted a gynaecologist in January 1976. He prescribed clomiphene citrate and also advised them to refrain from intercourse in the first two weeks of Mrs. R's menstrual cycle. When she noted a rise in her waking temperature, they were to have intercourse at 18 to 24-hourly intervals if possible. Mrs. R developed cycle-related mood swings, being euphoric at ovulation time and irritable or depressed premenstrually.

Mrs. R became anorgasmic with intercourse and encouraged her husband to ejaculate as soon as possible. 'It was too mechanical, not making love for two weeks and then going at it like rabbits'.

In October 1976, Mrs. R had a laparoscopy, which was normal.

In June 1977 Mrs. R. became pregnant, but in October was diagnosed as having a hydatidiform mole. Her gynaecologist removed the mole vaginally and performed a dilation and curettage a week later. The couple were advised to use condoms or spermicide as contraception and Mrs. R's hormone levels were monitored. After about a year, she was again prescribed clomiphene citrate.

After six clomiphene courses, the gynaecologist suggested a postcoital test. Mrs. R, who attended alone, asked the nurse who carried out the test if any live sperm were present. 'No. It looks as if your vaginal fluids are killing them off'.

Mr. R was than asked to provide a semen specimen, which showed a very low sperm count. He was referred to a urologist who diagnosed a varicocoel and operated.

In January 1980, Mrs. R became pregnant and delivered a full-term healthy child.

Mr. R. was anxious to have more children and clomiphene citrate was re-instated.

Two years later, the sexual side of the marriage had deteriorated badly. Mrs. R. professed to enjoy sexual relations only when there was no chance of pregnancy. Her husband found this attitude strange and disturbing.

continued on p. 64

> **BOX 6G** (continued)
>
> In January 1986 the gynaecologist referred them to an endocrinologist. He ordered a hysterosalpingogram and a further laparoscopy. As Mr. R's sperm count was again very low, he put Mrs. R on a course of Pergonal and Prophasyl. The programme involved daily injections, mid-cycle daily blood scans and mid-cycle daily ultrasounds.
>
> When she menstruated at the end of the first treatment cycle, Mrs. R declined to continue treatment. She was a solicitor and had the time-demands of a big case coming to court shortly. The recriminations that followed led up to divorce proceedings.

so given the wide publicity currently given to procedures such as the *in vitro* fertilisation programme. Patients present with the belief that the problem can probably be fixed, and some are going to be disappointed.

The case history in Box 6G is rather long. We thought it worthwhile to include it because it illustrates many points relevant to infertility treatment and counselling:

- Extensive investigations were carried out.
- Time-consuming and uncomfortable procedures were involved.
- The cost of some procedures and medications was not covered by Medibank, Medicare or the couple's private health fund.
- The investigations originally focussed on one partner alone.
- Not only were the couple not offered supportive counselling, they never felt that they had been given **permission** to discuss sexual matters.
- The interventions and their impact on the couple's relationship appeared to be a major factor in the subsequent marriage breakdown.

How to be supportive

When a patient or couple who have been having unprotected intercourse for a year or more without a pregnancy present, take a sexual history at once. If a patient presents alone, ask to see the partner and suggest that they try to attend together whenever possible.

There are good reasons for this:

- It emphasises that it is a shared problem. Both partners will be under similar stress.

- You will need to investigate both partners physically. In cases where a physical cause is found, it is about 60% a female problem, 40% male.[12]
- Both partners may need counselling if problems arise. It is helpful to have an ongoing relationship with them.

Before embarking on any investigations, tell the couple honestly what they are to expect. A simple solution may be found in a short time. On the other hand the investigations and treatment procedures may be prolonged, expensive, time-consuming, uncomfortable or embarrassing.

Right at the beginning, it is important to find out if both partners are equally as keen to achieve a pregnancy. Be aware that this may change, especially if interventions are focused on one partner alone.

As far as possible, couples should be encouraged to make only minimal changes in frequency of intercourse. Even so, many people respond, as Mrs. R. did, with the feeling that they have changed from a sexual person in their own right into a baby-making machine.

At all sessions, the practitioner should ask if the investigations and interventions are affecting the couple's sex life. A good preamble is, 'Some people find that this kind of treatment takes the spontaneity out of sex and makes it rather mechanical. Has that bothered either of you at all?' If it has, you can make a cost-benefit analysis of the relative values of continuing with treatment or taking a few months off.

Another issue to be addressed is the feeling of failure when the woman does not conceive. 'I cry every month when I see the blood on the toilet paper'. The practitioner can encourage patients to talk about this and be alert for any blaming going on in the relationship.

Of course, the fact that many Australian couples, especially those of higher socioeconomic status, are delaying starting a family until several years after marriage puts an additional stress on them when a fertility problem arises. There is the feeling that the woman's reproductive time is running out.

There are some important considerations when the treatment is deemed to be unsuccessful and terminated. If **you** decide to end treatment, the couple may be angry, distressed or feel abandoned. It is vital to introduce the topic of termination tentatively and perhaps be prepared to continue for a while, with a specified time limit. If the patients themselves decide to discontinue, it's very easy to feel angry yourself about the time and expertise you have invested in their case. Try to ask a non-judgemental open-ended question such as, 'What are your reasons for wanting to stop now?' This format avoids the confrontational 'Why?' and obliquely implies that they may wish to resume treatment at some future date. Partnership discord is a rather common factor in withdrawing from infertility treatment. Be alert for it and prepared to offer counselling or refer if necessary.

Finally, do not assume that the end of treatment implies the end of the couple's need for support. Many people feel a very real sense of bereavement when they have to abandon their hopes for a child and may continue to need help. In some cases, termination of treatment may represent a unilateral decision by one or other partner and be a potent source of partnership discord, as illustrated by our case history.

Linda Salzer's[13] book is a valuable source of insights into the psychological aspects of infertility.

References

1. Annon, J.S and Robinson, C.H. The use of vicarious learning models in treatment of sexual concerns. In J. LoPiccolo and L. LoPiccolo (eds) *Handbook of sex therapy*. New York: Plenum Press, 1978: 35–56.
2. Masters, W.H and Johnson, V.E. *Human sexual inadequacy*. Boston: Little, Brown and Company, 1970.
3. Kaplan, H.S. *The new sex therapy*. New York: Brunner/Mazel, 1974.
4. Kinsey, A.C, Pomeroy, W.B, Martin, C.E. *Sexual behaviour in the human male*. Philadelphia: W.B. Saunders, 1948.
5. Comfort, A. *The joy of sex. A gourmet guide*. London: Mitchell Beazley, 1987.
6. White, E and Silverstein, C. *The joy of gay sex: an intimate guide for gay men to the pleasures of a gay lifestyle*. New York: Simon and Schuster, 1977.
7. Kinsey, A.C, Pomeroy, W.B, Martin, C.E and Gebhard, P.H. *Sexual Behavior in the human female*. Philadelphia: W.B. Saunders, 1953.
8. Loulan, J. *Lesbian sex*. San Francisco: Spinsters/Aunt Lute, 1984.
9. Loulan, J. *Lesbian passion. Loving ourselves and each other*. San Francisco: Spinsters/Aunt Lute, 1987.
10. Goldberg, G. Suggestion as a general structure and a specific strategy in the behavioural treatment of vaginismus. *Australian Journal of Clinical and Experimental Hypnosis*, 1983: 11, 39–47.
11. Munjack, D.J and Oziel, *Sexual medicine and counseling in office practice: a comprehensive treatment guide*. Boston: Little, Brown and Company, 1980.
12. Hensleigh, P. Infertility. In M.U. Barnard, B.J. Clancy and K.E. Kramtz (eds) *Human sexuality for health professionals*. Philadelphia: W.B. Saunders, 1978.
13. Salzer, L. *Surviving infertility: a compassionate guide through the emotional crisis of infertility*. New York: Harper Perennial, 1991.
14. Semans, J.H. Premature ejaculation. A new approach. *South Med J*, 1956: 49, 353.
15. Wolpe, J and Lazarus, A.A. *Behaviour therapy techniques. A guide to the treatment of neuroses*. Oxford: Pergamon Press, 1966.

CHAPTER 7

REACTIONS TO STD INFECTION AND STD COUNSELLING

There are a number of reasons why counselling is an integral part of treating patients with STDs. First, the management of the illness, and the prevention of further infection of others or reinfection, is based on a number of behaviours which may be positively influenced by counselling. These include compliance with medication, cessation of unsafe sexual behaviour and other actions likely to transmit pathogens, and alteration of current and future sexual behaviour to prevent reinfection after treatment.

Second, STDs are set aside from most other conditions as being stigmatising — indeed, even talking about sexual behaviour, let alone about contracting a STD, causes difficulty to many medical practitioners and some health practitioners. In the case of widely publicised STDs, such as HIV infection and herpes, the stigmatisation is sufficiently severe as to lead to overt discrimination. The degree of stigmatisation may lead to psychological harm, including depression, loss of self-esteem, or anxiety, as well as loss of social supports.

While important in themselves, these factors in turn are likely to influence compliance with medication and other behavioural requirements for successful treatment.

The goals of STD counselling

Counselling is a vague term which is loosely applied in health practice and is sometimes used synonymously with 'talking'. Harris and Ramsay[1] comment that counselling is never aimless talking, but rather is a clear and coherent option for defining a problem, suitable for use from the first contact with a patient. There are a number of goals specific to STD counselling.

Providing comprehensive care
The goal of counselling is to assist the practitioner to provide comprehensive and thorough care for the patient. It must never be a

substitute for treating the illness, but rather should assist in history-taking, management, compliance with treatment, and prevention of future infection, as well as identification of associated psychosocial difficulties which may not have been evident initially.

Providing information

Counselling should include provision of specific information to the patient which will help them to understand the condition, its management, and prevent recurrence. This is often referred to as 'education' and should be aimed at preventing spread of disease or reinfection. This is set out in detail in the chapter on pre- and post-test counselling.

Reducing psychological sequelae

A degree of psychological harm, usually acute but occasionally chronic, may come from the knowledge of having a socially stigmatised condition. This may range from the feeling of being 'punished' for sexual activity, to loss of self-esteem from the contraction of an unacceptable illness, to the effects of making others (such as spouse or partner) aware that their partner has had sexual contact outside a primary relationship. This latter result of an STD may itself include sequelae such as relationship breakdown, depression or anxiety, or extreme and dysfunctional guilt.

Informing the partner(s)

With many STDs, it is advisable that contact tracing or partner notification, and concurrent management of partners occur both to prevent patient reinfection, and to prevent further spread of the particular disease. This sensitive area of patient management needs careful explanation as patients are often initially reluctant to contact partners. Where both partners are being simultaneously treated by the practitioner, relationship counselling may often need to occur as a function of one patient blaming the other for the STD or because the exposure of outside sexual contact leads to strains in the relationship.

The counselling process in STD management

The counselling process can be easily followed by most medical practitioners, regardless of whether they have had specific training in counselling. It requires only clear goals, a warm manner, and an understanding of the issues and processes involved. Probably the most important starting point is to give the patient an opportunity to express discomfort and the practitioner to recognise this discomfort. Most patients have usually thought quite a lot about the issues before they consult a practitioner, and often have arrived at some conclusions about the nature of their problems. However, there are a number of special issues which emerge in STD and AIDS counselling which need to be addressed.

The meaning of STD to the individual

Little of a scientific nature has been written about the meaning of STD infection to the individual, and little empirical research has been carried out on this area. This chapter attempts to explain the **beliefs** underlying psychological reactions to STDs and the reasons for psychological problems and approaches to counselling them when they occur.

In discussing the meaning of STDs to the individual, there appear to be at least five separate attributions.

1. STDs are a deserved outcome of indiscriminate sexual behaviour and punishment for sexual sins.
2. STDs are a consequence of individual inadequacy that leads to sexually indiscriminate behaviour.
3. STDs are a consequence of a breakdown in traditional social values and rapid social change.
4. STDs are the result of an individual coming into intimate contact with a virulent pathogen.
5. STDs are a sign of being sexually active and a matter of pride.

Note that there is a hierarchy of blame from attribution 1 to attribution 5. This parallels a similar hierarchy of the degree to which the individuals see themselves responsible for the infection. However, it is important to recognize that different models will apply in different cultures, and will depend on the degree to which there is a psychological investment in sexual behaviour.

Equally important, the meaning of STDS to the patient and to a lesser degree to the health practitioner will affect not only the compliance with treatment, but also the psychological response to infection and probably the subsequent risks of exposure to STDs the patient takes. Diagnosing the psychological difficulties surrounding STDs will be made easier if the practitioner is able to place the patient somewhere on a continuum so that they can understand the patient's perspective of the problem. The counselling approach will depend on which perspective the patient takes.

STD as punishment

When the individual sees the STD as punishment, a particularly religious background or never having come to terms with sexuality is common. In the case of the homosexual man, the individual will probably be at one of the first three stages of homosexual adjustment described by Cass,[6] in which their sexual orientation is not usually publicly acknowledged and almost invariably not accepted. Cass's stages are 1) Identity confusion; 2) Identity comparison; 3) Identity tolerance; 4) Identity acceptance; 5) Identity pride; and 6) Identity synthesis. The combination of the stigma of STD along with the stigma of homosexuality is an extremely powerful one, and the homosexual STD patient who sees his infection as an indication that he is being punished will need careful attention. The result of infection is likely to include remorse or sometimes clinical or subclinical depression as the individual is faced with the evidence of a sexual behaviour that he has probably compartmentalised or denied. This applies equally well to heterosexual people who have not accepted that sexual behaviour has occurred, or has occurred outside a primary relationship. There may also be anxiety about discovery or exposure. In such cases the anxiety or embarrassment may lead to defaulting from treatment, or denial of a homosexual orientation (or heterosexual contact outside a primary relationship) in the first place. Ross[2] has noted that a significant percentage of STD clinic attenders who are homosexual deny their sexual orientation to the attending practitioner, and that these individuals are most likely to expect the most negative reactions to their sexuality from others.

Such individuals who deny homosexual or extramarital contact are also most likely to be first attenders, and those who attend private practitioners rather than public clinics, may tend to deny their sexuality to a greater extent. It is important that the practitioner does not accept or reinforce the patient's negative view of their sexuality, particularly as this may be one of the first times the patient has admitted their sexual orientation or contacts to anyone outside of a small circle. Sometimes patients have apparently accepted their sexuality in the past but return to the first and most negative attribution of blame when they contract one of the more severe STDS: as an example, some people with AIDS or herpes who have been living openly homosexual (or 'fast lane' heterosexual) lives have seen their disease as a 'punishment from God' and blamed it on their sexuality. In some cases this may also be associated with an increase in religiosity in a person with AIDS. The combination of sexuality and STDs is a psychologically powerful one, and for the patient's mental well-being, if it is apparent that they see their STD infection as a 'punishment', assessment of the need for reassurance or correction must be made. The situation is more difficult if this is part of the patient's 'acceptance' of AIDS and/or death. In such cases, it is helpful to have access to accepting clergy for referral.

Venereophobias and the 'worried well'

This first category of the meaning of infection to the individual is most notable for its mental health consequences, which in many cases require more attention than the STD. Venereophobia, which is discussed below, in which there is no evidence of STD infection but the patient is convinced that infection has occurred, most commonly occurs in patients who see it as punishment for some real or imagined misdeed, usually of a sexual nature. The attention given to HIV infection and AIDS in the past few years has made 'AIDS phobias' a reasonably common clinical phenomenon in venereology, with the individuals presenting usually being concerned over sexual contact outside of primary relationships, and experiencing stress at work or in relationships which often acts as a trigger. Ross[3] has suggested that by providing the patient with insight into the additional factors which have led them to present with this concern at this time, the issue of HIV infection will often drop away and the other concerns (guilt over sexual behaviour or outside sexual relationships for which the possibility of HIV infection is 'punishment') will emerge.

BOX 7

Aids phobia

Mr C, a 25-year-old waiter, presented on referral from a hospital physician. He had been convinced he had AIDS for the past 3 weeks. While he had been living in a heterosexual relationship for the past 4 years, his partner had become pregnant 3 months previously. The sole risk factors for HIV infection were two homosexual encounters (all insertor fellatio) in the past year, one in Australia and one in southern Europe. He had subsequently avoided any further homosexual enounters from fear of contracting AIDS.

Symptoms on presentation included mild unilateral cervical lymphadenopathy, arthralgia, fatigue and insomnia, and suicidal ideation associated with the thought that he was going to die of AIDS.

> **BOX 7**
> (cont.)
> Mr C had had hepatitis A one year previously and had convinced himself this was cancer: three years previously he had convinced himself he had herpes following another homosexual encounter. Apart from severe psoriasis from the age of 17, there was no history of medical or psychiatric illness.
>
> Mr C's attitudes to homosexuality were negative: he stated that he had no emotional attraction to males, had homosexual encounters only for the physical pleasure, and was as hurtful as possible in rejecting those who had fellated him. As an adolescent he had actively encouraged his peers to attack homosexual men, and he now saw AIDS as 'God's judgement on homosexuals'.
>
> Four weeks previously, Mr C had completed a course of hypnotherapy, in which he had talked about his homosexual activities and his guilt over them for the first time, and been advised that there was no reason to punish himself over this. On presentation his DSM-III axis I diagnosis was hypochondriasis (300-70) and his belief that he had AIDS was of delusional quality.
>
> Two sessions of interpretive psychotherapy and a negative confirmatory HIV antibody test result (which Mr C would not initially believe) enabled him to see the relationship between his previous beliefs that he had cancer or herpes and his present belief he had AIDS. His insight into the dynamics of his disease conviction suggested it was not delusional as initially suspected. He was also able to recognize that the surfacing of the issue of his homosexual behavior during hypnotherapy had apparently forced his denial of his bisexuality toward affective discharge, and the subsequent decompensation had resulted in his belief that he had AIDS as a 'punishment'. A further contributor was the ambivalence he felt over his partner's pregnancy and his uncertainty over marriage and settling down. On follow-up three months later, Mr C admitted to still occasionally thinking about AIDS but these thoughts were not intrusive and he was trying to avoid homosexual encounters to reduce dissonance between his sexual attitudes and activities. His arthralgia and fatigue had been further investigated and a diagnosis of rheumatoid arthritis was subsequently made.

Brief insight-oriented counselling is the treatment of choice provided there is no evidence of psychosis, but it is important not to perform repeated HIV testing which may only reinforce the patient's conviction of infection. Paradoxical interventions[4] have been suggested as appropriate to psychotherapy with people with intractable AIDS worry, but these interventions (which involve treating the individual as if they were infected in order to release then from their rigid and distressing beliefs) should be carried out only by trained psychotherapists.

STDs as evidence of maladjustment

This second category has much in common with the first category in which STDs are seen as a punishment. While the reason for the individual's dysphoria on realizing that they have an STD may be a result of lack of acceptance of their sexual orientation, the basis is not religious and the discomfort not so pronounced. Nevertheless, the major difficulties are also likely to be psychological, but denial through keeping sexual orientation separate from other aspects of their life may also be present. Married men frequently fall into this category, and their homosexual activities are thus more likely to occur in public toilets to avoid the need for emotional contact with a partner. (Humphreys[5] found that over half of men who had sex in public toilets were married). As a result, the contacts are often likely to be unknown, and there is the added complication that the patient's wife may have been infected, and be unaware of her spouse's bisexuality. Since a sizeable proportion of homosexual men (between 10 and 20 percent) marry, and since those who marry are usually those less accepting of their homosexuality,[6] such people may be frequently represented in those with sexual orientation dysphorias. A comparable situation will occur in the case of the person who has had extramarital contact.

In contrast to situations where individuals are unhappy at being homosexual (or at having affairs outside a primary relationship or frequent sexual contacts), however, such patients become disturbed by their sexuality only when it produces negative consequences such as STD infection. The advent of AIDS has also produced a marked increase in patients falling into this category in the past few years.

A second group within this category are those with mild discomfort with a treatable STD infection, and who recognise that there is nothing they can do about their sexual behaviour but feel that it might be easier to be monogamous (or heterosexual). They rarely present a problem in terms of either compliance with treatment or mental state. On the other hand, too great a degree of discomfort may result in sexual contacts that are anonymous because for some people known partners and emotional contact could be too guilt-engendering. Contact tracing is thus likely to be difficult, although returning for proof of cure is usually not a problem. Treatment of this attributional group is similar to that of the first group if 'AIDS phobias' arise, and may require psychotherapy.

STDs as the fault of a sick society

In this group, the blame for STD infection is likely to be projected toward others rather than internalised, and the individual, if homosexual, is most likely to be at Cass's[7] fifth stage of homosexual development. The fifth stage, according to Cass, is the period where the individual accepts his homosexuality and defines his whole lifestyle in terms of it. Thus, to the extent where he allocates blame for STD infection, it cannot lie with his sexual orientation, which is so centrally important to him, but must lie elsewhere. Elsewhere is usually the society that so stigmatises homosexuals that it may be necessary (although much less so than in the past) to meet in secluded places and keep sexual contacts concealed.

Stigmatisation may also affect the number of sexual partners by lowering self-esteem to the point where relationships are not possible, and either multiple partners or no partners may be the adjustment sought to counter a negative self-image. While these arguments are based on reality in places where sexuality is severely stigmatised and legal penalties are also severe, or in rural areas or small towns, they appear to seldom apply to those whose sexuality (particularly homosexuality) is the central defining construct of their lifestyle. Essentially, those who believe that STDs are the fault of a discriminatory society are unable to accept that any fault lies with them, and may be less responsive to suggestions about cutting down at-risk practices. In some cases, such a suggestion will be construed as a condemnation of their sexuality, and the consultation terminated. In others, STD infection becomes a matter of pride, indicating emancipation from the perceived restrictive and conservative sexual habits of monogamy and 'ownership' of sexual partners. Where sexual behaviour is seen as a political or social statement, it is less likely that it will be open to modification.

Similarly, where an individual has 'come out' recently as a homosexual or become recently heterosexually active, it is most likely that there will be more frequent sexual contacts both in response to a previous lack of sexual contact in most cases, and because public understanding of homo- and heterosexuality centres on their sexual component rather than their emotional or social component. In such cases, sexual activity may be higher than it would otherwise be due to an affirmation of the individual's core identity. If this is the case, then suggestions that attempt to modify sexual behaviour could be seen as a rejection of their sexuality, and thus the point should be cautiously approached. If, however, this does not appear to be occurring after a lapse of several years, it may be advisable to raise the issue by determining the meaning of sexual behaviour to the patient and by attempting to identify any personal difficulties that may be driving their sexual behaviour. Generally, this stage is the opposite of the STD as 'punishment group', in that the latter see their sexuality as inviting retribution while the former see their sexuality as a central, defining and positive aspect of their lifestyle.

STDs as just another infection

For some people, STD infection is not highly emotionally laden and carries no investment. Such individuals are likely, if homosexual, to be in Cass's stage 5 or stage 6, in which a homosexual orientation is seen as being only one of many identifications the individual has, and not central to identity or lifestyle. Of course, STD infection (HIV and herpes excepted) **is** medically just another curable infection with varying risks associated, but few people are able to see it that way. In terms of dealing with individuals at this stage of STD perception, there is little problem in making suggestions of modification of at-risk behaviours, but on the other hand if infection does not cause psychological distress, there is little reason to do so unless the risk is a major one and incurable (such as with hepatitis B or C, or HIV) or the effects are long-term (such as herpes).

People who have this attribution of the cause of STDs tend to have identified themselves as actively heterosexual or as homosexual for a longer period and approach sexuality in a fairly hedonistic way. Thus, if modification to partner numbers as a response to AIDS or other STDs is necessary, partner numbers may be cut down without great psychological trauma. However, if partner numbers are important to the person to maintain self-esteem, then that individual may externalise the blame and see STDs as the 'fault of a sick society'.

STDs as a source of pride

In some situations, particularly with adolescents who are eager to demonstrate their maturity by demonstrating sexual conquest or desirability, STDs may be a source of pride. In such a situation, it will be difficult to suggest preventive measures since they may diminish the individual's identity as adult or sexually desirable and threaten one of their sources of self esteem. Such individuals may also fall into the fifth stage, 'identity pride', of Cass's model, and may see attempts to reduce the chances of reoccurrence (although not cure of individual episodes) as diminishing what may be perceived as a mark of prestige among peers. With the advent of AIDS, however, it is to be hoped that this attitude will become less common. It may be possible to invest condom use with some of the positive properties of STDs in this attribution as a preventive strategy.

Counselling

In counselling, the aim of practitioners should be to remove the psychological involvement to the point where STDs are just another infectious disease. However, the attendant consequence is to also remove the pressures, positive and negative, on individuals to modify their behaviours. Pressure to modify behaviour will thus be a consequence of the risks that STDs carry (for example, high risk for HIV and herpes, lower for gonorrhoea).

It is hard to describe a general approach to counselling for STDs because each patient will come with an individual background and context of infection. However, the goal of counselling is to have the patient accept that STD infection is not a punishment, but is a medical condition which needs to be taken seriously and avoided in future. Further, it needs to be emphasised that STD infection can be avoided without necessarily making major changes in lifestyle. Often, an appropriate context for counselling can be achieved by letting the patient see that the practitioner does not share the pessimistic or the boastful view about STDs which is held by the patient. Counselling is nevertheless a means to an end rather than an end in itself, and the specific content of the counselling will depend on the specific issue raised.

Dealing with psychological problems

At the point where the practitioner has assessed where the patient falls on the continuum of response to STD infection, problems may emerge which have to be dealt with. Patients who see STDs as an indication of inadequacy or as a punishment may exhibit distress or disgust. It is important that the practitioner does not reinforce such feelings, as this will only add to the distress, and will have little effect on modifying at-risk behaviours except to make them more guilt-ridden and the patient less likely to re-present. The counselling should focus on the patient's feelings initially, and once these have been clarified (by reflecting the practitioner's understanding back to the patient for confirmation), the focus should turn to the events or behaviours surrounding the distress or discomfort.

Setting goals for counselling

At this stage, it is important that there is agreement between the practitioner and the patient as to whether there is a problem and the nature of the problem, since counselling cannot proceed if there is no agreement, and goals for the counselling must be set. These goals may be as simple as checking that the patient understands the reasons for the maintenance of medication, or may extend to intermediate goals such as making sure the patient understands the need to use condoms, and either has access to them or has appropriate social skills to insist on using them. More complex goals may include understanding the reasons for compulsive sexual behaviour, marital or relationship counselling, coming to terms with a homosexual or bisexual orientation, or decreasing guilt, anxiety or depression following a sexual encounter. In some cases, the practitioner may choose to refer the patient on to a colleague with greater experience in the area.

Without summarising in detail the many issues which STD infection may elicit or precipitate, it is important to note two points. First, the practitioner will probably be the only individual with whom the patient will be able to discuss the infection (and thus fulfils an important role as a supportive listener for a wide range of conflicts and concerns). Second, as already noted, the stigmatisation surrounding STDs may precipitate a number of dysphoric mood states or identity or relationship crises which will require identification and management as much as the infection itself.

Practitioner Reactions to STDs

However, patients are not the only ones with beliefs about STDs. Each of the five stages described can also be used to describe practitioner attitudes to STD infection. Those who have read widely on the subject will be able to classify various authors and authorities on a continuum from seeing gonococci as 'God's little helpers' through to approaching them as just a part of infectious disease management. The important thing to note is that our attitudes as practitioners will affect our approach to our patients, and that our personal attitudes will interact with those of our patients. The consequence of this for behaviour modification of risky behaviours is enormous: to give two examples, the practitioner whose attributions of STDs are at the first level will discourage avoidance of risks because the 'punishment' is preordained and presumably unavoidable. Nor will any distinction be made between safe and unsafe sexual acts because the 'punishment' is seen as being for sexual activity, not particular specific sexual acts! On the other hand, the practitioner who believes Attribution 4 that sexuality is important and that STDs are just another infection may well have, as noted above, removed the pressures on individuals to modify their behaviours. This is particularly dangerous where practitioners see sexual contact in ideological terms and feel that to urge patients to decrease sexual partner numbers is tantamount to rejection of a particular mode of sexual expression.

The interaction between patients and practitioners who hold conflicting attributions for STDs may also lead to tension, anger, transference and countertransference issues and resistance to taking advice or treatment, particularly where more divergent attributions are held. It is critical to ascertain one's own position and make some estimate of the position of one's patient before trying to educate, or to modify risky behaviours.

Genital herpes infections and counselling

Herpes simplex infection of the genital region falls midway in its implications and impact between the essentially curable bacterial STDs and HIV. While herpes is not a fatal infection there is no cure although treatment for individual episodes is available. However, counselling with herpes is particularly important because there has been some suggestion that recurrent viral infection may be influenced by psychological factors.

Linking psychological status and recurrence: The recurrence of herpes simplex virus (HSV) disease has been linked with both psychological and physiological factors.

Drob and colleagues[8] noted that lack of social skills, including assertiveness, and inability to vent emotions may be associated with recurrences, and Goldmeir[9] has linked non-psychotic psychological states, such as anxiety and obsessiveness, to high frequencies of recurrence. Psychotherapy has been shown to reduce frequency of herpes episodes, and over three quarters of people with HSV regarded stress as a major factor in their recurrence. Further, the stress of having HSV was felt to prime new recurrences. Thus it is important to note that there may be a link between psychological state and recurrence, and to attempt to break that nexus or to reduce the stressors.

***Effects on lifestyle*:**   The impact of HSV infection upon significant life areas should not be underestimated. Drob and colleagues[8] found that the majority of people with genital HSV reported that infection and concern about recurrence made them less capable of physical warmth and intimacy, they enjoy sex less, and feel less sexually desirable. All the patients in Drob's study found that work performance was hampered. It is important to ascertain the specific effects of the infection (or concern about the infection) on significant life areas and to acknowledge these as a possible focus for intervention. In the same study, a majority of those surveyed reported disturbance of affect (feeling that herpes is incompatible with happiness, and being pessimistic about the future course of the illness) and Drob and colleagues also note that in an earlier survey conducted by the American Social Health Association, 84% of people with genital herpes also reported depression.

Sexual dysfunction: Both studies reported above found that genital herpes infection had sexual consequences. Such consequences included reduced interest in sex, lowered ability to achieve orgasm, avoidance of intimacy, and less enjoyment of sex when it did occur. This is probably associated with feeling less sexually desirable because of herpes (reported by over two thirds of respondents), and feeling repugnant to others.

***Providing psychological support*:**   Interpersonal relations may also be affected by the infection or, more frequently, concern about its effect on relationships if it is generally known that one is infected. Aral and colleagues[10] report that over 30% of Americans say that they would not asociate with someone who has herpes, and Drob and colleagues[8] also noted that the majority of their patients felt thay would not be accepted by others if their herpes infection became known. In the same study, the lack of social support from others in dealing with herpes was also seen as a major problem, as was being prevented from getting to know people to whom one is sexually attracted. In this sort of situation, it is important that the practitioner be prepared to provide psychological support as well as professional advice.

Managing altered affect: Affect may also be altered by infection — the degree to which this may be physical ('post-viral depression') or psychological is not known. Nevertheless, the alteration may be sufficiently profound to consider anxiolytic or antidepressant medication in some cases. The most common concerns expressed by those with HSV infection include concern about infecting others, recurrence and the future course of the illness, and sometimes self-destructive feelings.

These general guidelines for counselling are based on the situation of chronic recurrent viral infections such as herpes, but generally apply to similar infections. There are more similarities than differences with herpes and recently diagnosed HIV infection and what is true about herpes will also be true for HIV (and vice-versa). However, reactions to herpes will generally be less severe than to HIV. Nevertheless, experience in the psychological responses and counselling people with herpes has tended to focus on heterosexual individuals, while to date the HIV literature has focused on homosexual men.

Staging of reactions to HIV and AIDS

Just as there are stages of reaction to attributions for STD infection, there are stages through which individuals may pass when infected with AIDS or other STDs. The case of AIDS is the most clearly defined, given the major traumas associated with a potentially fatal sexually transmissible infection. In many ways these are similar to the model of stages of coming to terms with terminal illness described by Kübler-Ross[9] but also differ in some important respects since the trauma is often the stigmatisation rather than the possibility of death. These reactions are more marked the lower one goes down the attributional scale. It is important to realize that the emotional impact of telling an individual that they have HIV infection is not significantly different to that of telling them they have full AIDS. Rosser and Ross,[12] in a two-country study of homosexual men, found that the emotional distress of being informed one was HIV seropositive, had an AIDS-related complex, or had full AIDS was judged to be of the same emotional magnitude, although the amount of life change judged to be associated with these diagnoses was significantly different. Further, the emotional impact of HIV infection appears to be qualitatively and quantitatively different from that of curable STDs. Rosser and Ross[12] also found that emotional distress from receiving a positive HIV antibody test was not significantly different from that caused by a diagnosis of AIDS or HIV disease, and also from the diagnosis of AIDS in a lover or the death of a lover. Those who were HIV seropositive, moreover, evaluated life events as having a greater emotional impact than those uninfected, suggesting that HIV seropositive status increases the perceived stress of life events. These data suggest that non-curable or possibly fatal STDs may elicit reactions which are different in both quality and degree from potentially curable STDs.

Ross, Tebble and Viliunas[13] have described the reactions of homosexual men to asymptomatic HIV infection. These psychological stages and the clinical issues associated with such stages are summarised below. They note that HIV infection may not lead to death for a proportion of individuals and thus the Kübler-Ross model of acceptance of terminal illness is frequently inappropriate, particularly if as is believed, cofactors may influence progression of HIV infection. There is in addition considerable stigma attached to infection and this stigmatised status is not usually visible or identifiable. In this regard the model is appropriate to herpes infection as well. Also for this reason, the model contains some similarities to models of homosexual identity formation. This is to be expected, since a significant proportion of individuals carrying antibodies to HIV in the western world are homosexual or bisexual men. In many cases they will use a previously appropriate and successful model to manage a second stigmatised status such as HIV infection. The degree of clinical utility of the model, Ross, Tebble and Viliunas stress must, however, be determined by further research. They note that this model, while staged, is fluid (allowing for regression as well as progression) and that some individuals may neither experience every stage nor progress beyond particular stages.

Stages 1 and 2 — shock, denial and anger: The initial stage describes the common reactions to major unanticipated trauma. Denial may operate as defence to prevent decompensation, but the psychological processes operating commonly include guilt at being responsible for infection, anger at self or those perceived responsible for infection, and powerlessness associated with lack of control or knowledge of outcome.

This is exacerbated by associated minority status (further stigmatisation within and beyond an already stigmatised group).

Stage 3 — withdrawal: This stage describes the response to recognition that one has an infection which may lead to isolation, either imposed or self-imposed, sexual or social. Recognition of the associated stigma activates previously useful stigma management models, particularly those in use in groups such as homosexuals and injecting drug users whose status, like that of the HIV antibody-positive individuals or people with herpes virus infection, is concealable. Individuals in this stage tend to keep to themselves as part of their uncertainty about the reactions of others. A significant component of this keeping to themselves may be related to fear of infecting others and to depression.

Stage 4 — bargaining (substage 4A — 'coming out' to significant others): Stage 4A follows at this point not the Kübler-Ross model of terminal illness but more closely the Cass model of stages of homosexual identity formation. Disclosing one's positive HIV antibody or herpes infection status to certain carefully selected individuals follows the process of disclosure to individuals who are most likely to be accepting or who are family or significant others. Psychological processes include bargaining with society (through those disclosed to) over acceptance, expression of the need to still be loved, and displacement of stress on to others. The form of the reaction of others will determine the presenting problems, but these commonly include coping with stress related to disclosure, rejection, and confrontation. If those disclosed to were unaware of the previous stigmatised status, reactions tend to be more consistently negative.

Substage 4B — looking for others: This stage also has elements in common with acceptance of a stigmatised identity as described by Cass, particularly the seeking out of others in a similar situation. Processes involved include seeking positive reinforcement and the social and psychological support of others with whom one shares a common difficulty. Peer support provides confidence which comes with recognition of one's antibody-positive status and sharing of problems and reactions with those in a similar position. Difficulties which may emerge include dependency on HIV antibody-positive or herpes-infected peers, one's infection status becoming one's dominant identification to the exclusion of others, and loss of anonymity if one is identified with a stigmatised group.

Substage 4C — special status: This stage of herpes or HIV antibody-positive status acceptance is one we have noted is common in those individuals who have previously lacked a strong sense of identity. Those who have had no ambivalence about a previous stigmatised status such as a homosexual orientation may often proceed direct to substage 4D. Substage 4C turns alienation into an advantage (similar to the identity pride stage of Cass's model of homosexual identity formation) where individuals see themselves as something different and special, needed by others. Psychologically, this stage may also represent reaction formation or a sense of guilt or self blame over becoming infected, leading to action in substage 4D. Problems associated with this stage include over-identification with, and dependency on, one's 'special' status and splitting the world into an 'us and them' dichotomy. Self-help groups may foster such a status as a stage toward acceptance.

Substage 4D — altruistic behaviour: Altruistic behaviour connects the issues in substages 4B and 4C into action. There is a feeling of community and belonging within the stigmatised sub-group, and beyond this a desire to affirm that identity. The strong desire to give and share with others may be a part of the process of 'making friends with one's disease' taken to the point of acceptance of a stigmatised status and denial of its stigma. The need to serve and in many cases to 'go public', though, can lead to problems of stigmatisation, burnout and over-reaction. However, this is balanced by provision of a purpose in a life which may have been disrupted by a diagnosis of HIV status or herpes, and provision of a mechanism with which to cope with this condition.

Stage 5 — acceptance: Most models, including those of Kübler-Ross and Cass, have a final acceptance of a perceived negative status or negative situation as their resolution. Logically, integration of herpes infection or positive HIV antibody status as part of one's identity should follow. This stage appears to be a balance between the altruism of substage 4D and attention to self. Problems which tend to present are resistance to further change of those behaviours which may place self or others at risk, and a degree of apathy over health status.

These stages are an approximation of the psychological processes operating in individuals who are HIV antibody positive or, to a lesser extent, have genital herpes. However, they do raise the issue of the normal progression of illness behaviours in individuals with STDs, and particularly the role of illness behaviours given that there is no possibility of secondary gain (except as exhibited in factitious illness such as factitious AIDS).

Abnormal illness behaviours in STDs

Little data are available on illness behaviour in STDs: it was generally assumed that illness behaviours in STDs were identical to those in other comparable illnesses. However, it has important implications for treatment. In the case of individuals with an erroneous conviction that they have an STD, which Hart[14] refers to as venereoneurosis, there is abnormal illness behaviour in terms of both general hypochondriasis and a strong disease conviction without demonstrable evidence of infection. There may also be an indication that the patient believes they 'deserve' the infection, as noted in the previous section of this chapter. In the case of other individuals, and perhaps more common, is the refusal to see STD as an illness but perhaps only as a minor non-significant risk of a particular lifestyle.

Clinical observation has tended to suggest that in the case of the absence of illness behaviour, patients may frequently compromise treatment by discontinuing medication after symptoms have resolved, continuing sexual activity after symptom resolution but before clearance, or not returning for proof of cure. Thus, both abnormal illness behaviour and lack of illness behaviour may have implications for the management of STDs.

Ross[15] looked at illness behaviours in STD clinic attenders, and found that contrary to expectations, it was the repeated attenders rather than the first attenders who displayed the greatest anxiety and hypochondriasis over STD infection. Those with higher previous numbers of infections also tended to deny life stresses more, and attribute their problems to the episode of illness. Such individuals also displayed symptom preoccupation, and higher levels of symptom exaggeration. In comparison, first attenders tended to deny that an STD was an illness, which would appear to be in some cases also a denial of the contraction of an often stigmatising illness. Compared to other illness behaviours, in which there may be substantial secondary gain from sympathy and assistance, STD infection appears to be quite different and to develop as a function of repeated infections. In such cases, it would appear that STD infection tends to be seen as a chance event until after several infections, when it is then seen not only as an illness but also as a result of particular behaviours.

In the same study, Ross also found that there were few differences in illness behaviour with STD infections between heterosexual and homosexual men, apart from the fact that there is a less negative reaction to STD infection in the gay community (probably as a result of the greater awareness of STDs in gay subcultures and the greater self-definition of homosexual men in sexual terms). It was also noted, using non-STD controls attending general practice and psychiatric outpatient clinics, that the STD clinic population was closer to the psychiatric population than the general practice one. This tends to confirm the finding of Catalan and colleagues that 40% of a United Kingdom STD clinic population had some degree of psychological disturbance on a screening test. It is unclear whether the disturbance was a function of having a stigmatised illness such as an STD or inherent in STD clinic attenders. There may be major differences between public and private clinics, and between the accuracy of admissions at STD clinics depending on individual factors such as practitioner approach and clinic environment.

Admission of details of sexuality

The picture that emerges of the variables predictive of whether the patient reveals a homosexual orientation (and, one might assume, other details about their sexuality) when presenting to a STD clinic or health practitioner is a coherent one. Nonadmitters are likely to conceal their sexuality or homosexuality from most people, to expect the most negative social reaction to their sexuality or homosexuality from significant others and society in general, and to believe in much more rigid and conservative behaviours as being appropriate for men and women. As compared with those who admit to homosexual contact, nonadmitters are also more likely to report themselves as having had no previous STDs. The nonadmitter thus emerges as an individual who expects particularly negative reactions to revealing his/her sexuality.

These data have a number of practical applications for counselling. A lack of previous sexually transmitted infections in nonadmitters suggests that the clinic situation will be a new and potentially frightening one, in which condemnation is expected: in subsequent visits to a clinic the patient will tend to be less apprehensive if the clinician's approach has been nonjudgemental. Thus, the first visit is crucial in building up the rapport which is so critical for taking sexual histories and sexual counselling. The apparent passivity and lack of assertion that are also predictors of failure to reveal matters about one's sexuality suggest that many patients may have trouble expressing what is construed as negative information that may elicit a negative response. It may also be that when clinicians take histories in a manner that implies that any sexual contact was a heterosexual or homosexual one, the patient may not have the courage to make a correction. However, these psychological factors will clearly operate in interaction with environmental factors such as the clinic, the clinician, and the legal and social climate regarding sexuality. Individual practitioners can do little more than to be aware of the factors operating, and seek to actively mitigate them through their interaction with patients, particularly emphasising genuineness and empathy as well as specifically dealing with their therapeutic acceptance of what patients may consider shameful or abnormal practices. The imposition of shame and guilt upon sexual interactions by religious and other traditional moralities is the single most important cause of psychological problems in STD treatment, and if the practitioner is able to assess and deal with this early in the treatment process, many difficulties may be prevented or minimised. Lack of consideration may even introduce or reinforce shame or guilt and produce an iatrogenically strengthened psychopathology. A high index of suspicion for psychosocial problems attendant on STD infection or reported infection is mandatory to ensure maximal compliance with treatment, contact tracing or partner notification, prevention and preventive education, and the possible contribution of psychosocial factors to relapse or reinfection should not be underestimated. It can, however, be to some extent neutralised by careful, sympathetic and tactful handling.

In conclusion, it can be demonstrated that psychological aspects of STDs play a central part in understanding their incidence, presentation, treatment and prevention. This is particularly true where the infection is not curable or associated with stigmatisation (such as genital herpes or HIV infection). In sexual counselling within the context of managing STDS, the psychological aspects of the problem may cause as much or more morbidity and distress as the physical ones, and these reactions need to be understood and treated by the practitioner. Understanding some of the stages and and ramifications of STDs (including HIV infection) which are described in this chapter, as well as some of the counselling approaches to them, should place the practitioner in a good position to deal with them in clinical practice.

References

1. Harris, R.D and Ramsay, A.T. *Health care counselling*. Sydney: Williams & Wilkins, 1988.
2. Ross, M.W. Psychosocial factors in admitting to homosexuality in sexually transmitted disease clinics. *Sex Transm Dis* 1985: 12, 83–86.
3. Ross, M.W. AIDS phobias: a report of four cases. *Psychopathology* 1988: 21, 26–30.
4. Salt, H, Miller, R, Perry L and Bor, R. Paradoxical interventions in counselling for people with intractable AIDS-worry. *AIDS Care*, 1989: 1, 38–44.
5. Humphreys, R.A.L. *Tearoom trade: a study of impersonal sex in public places*. London: Duckworth, 1970.
6. Ross, M.W. *The married homosexual man: a psychological study*. London: Routledge & Kegan Paul, 1983.
7. Cass, V.C. Homosexual identity formation: a theoretical model. *Journal of Homosexuality* 1979: 4, 219–235.
8. Drob, S, Leemer, L and Lifshutz, H. Genital herpes: the psychological consequences. *British Journal of Medical Psychology*, 1985: 58, 307–315.
9. Goldmeir, D. Psychosexual problems. *Br Med J* 1984: 288, 704–705.
10. Aral, S.O, Gates, W and Jenkins, W.C. Genital herpes: does knowledge lead to action? *Am J of Public Health*, 1985: 75, 69–71.
11. Kübler-Ross, E. *On death and dying*. London: Tavistock, 1969.
12. Rosser, B.R.S and Ross, M.W. Emotional and life change impact of AIDS on homosexual men in two countries. *Psychology and Health* 1988: 2, 301–317.
13. Ross, M.W, Tebble, W.E.M and Viliunas, D. Staging of reactions to AIDS virus infection in asymptomatic homosexual men. *Journal of Psychology and Human Sexuality* 1989: 2, 93–104.
14. Hart, G. *Sexual maladjustment and disease: an introduction to modern venereology*. Chicago: Nelson-Hall, 1977.
15. Ross, M.W. Illness behavior among patients attending a sexually transmitted disease clinic. *Sex Transm Dis* 1987: 14, 174–179.
16. Catalan J, Bradley, M, Gallwey, J and Hawton, K. Sexual dysfunction and psychiatric morbidity in patients attending a clinic for sexually transmitted diseases. *British Journal of Psychiatry* 1981: 138, 292–296.

CHAPTER 8

SEXUALITY AND PREVENTIVE HEALTH CARE

In modern medicine, the role of preventive health care is becoming increasingly important as individuals and communities express interest in maintaining some control over their health. The increase in knowledge about the antecedents of disease has also played a part in making preventive education possible, as has the increasing specialisation in health and the consequent emphasis on general practitioners and community health centres as being involved in the primary or secondary prevention of disease.

The major areas of sexuality in which prevention of difficulties may occur include contraception, Papanicolaou (pap) smears, and breast self-examination. Other areas which should also be considered should be the relationship of drugs to sexuality, testicular self-examination, and the dangers of some sex 'toys'. Of these areas, traditionally contraception and family planning is the most common.

Contraception

Health services have routinely advised on and prescribed contraception, particularly to women, and practice of this area of preventive sexual health is not controversial in the health care setting. As this has been extensively reviewed elsewhere[1] it will be briefly covered here.

There is no ideal method of contraception: each method has advantages and disadvantages, and contraception should be tailored to the case of the individual patient. Diamond[1] suggests that the role of the health practitioner is to make clear the relative advantages and disadvantages of each method in the light of the individual's age, health, and medical picture, as well as their social situation with regard to a partner, coital frequency and context, maturity, reliability (of both method and patient) and other relevant factors. Usually, contraception is a matter which is the concern of the woman and in taking any health history, the history of contraception will be included. It is a matter that should be raised in every case, and contraception should be reviewed from time to time to determine whether the method used is still the most appropriate if circumstances or medical knowledge change. Contraception is also a useful stepping off point to raise other areas of sexual preventive health.

Sexually transmissible disease prevention

The traditional way of preventing STDs has been the condom.[2] This is still the case. If male patients are sexually active with more than one partner, then condom use should be advised. While instructions are included with most condoms, the practitioner should assist the patient by discussing the major issues involved with the patient. These include using only water-based lubricant, as oil-based ones will perish the condom; expelling any air remaining in the teat of the condom when putting it on; ensuring that the condom covers the entire shaft of the penis but not the scrotum; and holding the condom in place during withdrawal. Because the adoption of safer sex practices has been shown to be greater where condoms have been provided at the site of counselling, practitioners may wish to consider offering condoms as part of STD counselling and education. This may do more to decrease the risk of STDs than any other single act the practitioner may perform.

One of the greatest difficulties in advising condom use is the negative attitudes held toward them by some people. Such negative attitudes include the view that it is 'like taking a shower in a raincoat' and the belief that they interrupt sexual pleasure and the sexual act. Many of these beliefs are based on the performance of the thicker rubber condoms of past decades (and are often voiced by people who have never used a condom). However, such apparent drawbacks as lessened sensitivity and interruption of sex may also be advantages. Lessened sensation may make the sexual act last longer. Integrating the placement of the condom into foreplay has also been reported as being extremely erotic. Generally, attitudes toward condoms are the greatest barrier to their use and the practitioner should be prepared to offer information which may change attitudes, as well as encouraging the use of, or providing a condom for experimentation.

While female condoms have been developed and trialled, at the time of writing they are not widely available but when they are, they should also be discussed with female patients on the same basis as the traditional condom is for male patients.

Prevention or early detection of cancer

The pap smear has been commonly used to detect cervical intra-epithelial neoplasia (CIN) which may develop, if untreated, into carcinoma in situ or disseminated carcinoma. The fact is that the great majority (40¢80%)[3] of cervical or vulvar higher grades of neoplasia involve human papilloma virus (HPV), the genital wart virus emphasises the need for both STD precautions as well as regular pap smears. The fact that almost all cases of CIN or carcinoma in situ can be successfully treated if detected early. Paavonen and colleagues[3] note that herpes simplex virus (HSV) has also been isolated from tumours of the lower genital tract, although the interactions between HPV and HSV are not fully understood.

From the perspective of preventive health, patients should be told of the relationship between sexually transmissible viruses and cancer of the lower genital tract. What should be emphasised is that by regular pap smears, almost all pre-cancerous abnormalities can be detected and successfully treated (usually on an outpatient basis). Unfortunately, many women are aware of the need for a regular annual pap smear but have no idea why they should have one. Simple and straightforward explanation of why people should take particular preventive precautions invariably increases the compliance rate considerably.

Genital warts may also be associated with cancers of other genital sites, most notably the anus and penis. While the risk of progression is significantly greater if there is immunosuppression, people who have had anal warts treated, and men with a history of penile warts, should be advised to reattend if there appears to be any recurrence. It is debatable whether explicit information on the possibility of malignancies should be provided given their low probability and the desire not to unduly scare people, but certainly the patient should be advised to have a high index of suspicion for regrowth and to attend if further abnormal growths are detected.

Pelvic inflammatory disease (PID) is usually caused by the migration of organisms from the vagina or cervix to the endometrium, fallopian tubes and (or) contiguous structures. It is a major cause of infertility as well as of acute or chronic abdominal pain. Weström and Mårdh[4] note that most cases of PID are caused by exogenous pathogens such as gonorrhoea or chlamydia. The link of STDs with PID is not well understood by many women, and again preventive education must be based on an understanding of what must be prevented and the possible health consequences of infection. Again, this is an area of health promotion which can be simply explained but very frequently is not. We cannot expect patients to take reasonable precautions until the reasons have been explained to them so that they may make an informed decision based on their own motivation rather than advice.

Most public STD clinics and health departments have a wide range of simple and easy to read material on STDs and their signs, consequences and avoidance or treatment, and if the practitioner is serious about preventive health services, these might be obtained either for display in the waiting room or distribution to patients.

Self-examination for cancers

Women

The best known example of self-examination for cancer is breast self-examination. However, it sometimes causes concern because women are unsure what to look for or what it might feel like, and because the subject of cancer is too frightening. Nevertheless, early detection of breast cancer will, all other things being equal, lead to an increased chance of successful treatment. Women who are at risk of breast cancer by reason of family history, not having had a pregnancy or having their first pregnancy later in life should be advised to regularly examine their breasts. While most lumps detected by breast self-examination prove to be benign, the advantages of early detection of those which prove to be malignant outweigh the disadvantages. Given that around one in ten women will have breast cancer, breast self-examination should be advised and explained to every female patient.

Where it is available, mammography is another service which will detect breast lumps at a size at which they are usually not detectable by self-examination, and this alternative should also be discussed with the patient where appropriate.

Men

Testicular cancer is the primary cause of cancer death in men between the ages of 15 and 34. However, it is also one of the most responsive to early treatment, with a success rate exceeding 90% for those without secondary spread.[5] Further, testicular self-examination is easily performed and any abnormalities usually quite easily detected. It is thus even more appropriate to advise as a preventive measure than breast self-examination for women. For some reason, however, it has been virtually ignored by health practitioners and by preventive health services. With male patients who are between adolescence and middle age, testicular self-examination should be advised and the reasons given. Where patients are at higher risk, for example having a history of an undescended testicle, such advice should be mandatory.

Sex toys

This category covers any object which can be inserted into the vagina, anus or urethra. While probably an uncommon practice, if patients present with injury which it is suspected may have been caused by insertion of a foreign object into an orifice then advice on the dangers of such practices is appropriate. Where there is definitive evidence, such as patients presenting with objects which cannot be extracted or which have caused injury, then obviously such advice is mandatory.

Where a patient derives sexual pleasure from insertion of objects, whether as part of sexual practice or as an aid to autoerotic practices, they will probably continue such activity. Thus it is important to suggest that if it is not possible to stop inserting objects, the objects should be unbreakable, without protrusions which cause trauma, and suitably lubricated. They should also have attachments which allow them to be retrieved. If patients do wish to continue the use of sex toys as part of their erotic repertoire, they should ensure that these toys are appropriate and safe.

Drugs

Drugs are frequently used in association with sexual contact, with alcohol probably being the most common. In the younger age group, so-called 'party drugs' (amphetamines and their derivatives) may also be used, and the use of volatile nitrites to enhance orgasm is common in some sections of the gay community. These drugs may be used simultaneously.

While drugs may have their own negative effects if taken in inappropriate doses, their prime risk with regard to sexual behaviour (see also the later chapter on drugs and sexual functioning) is to cloud judgement.

Where judgement is clouded, risks will be taken which would not normally be taken. Chief among these risks is having intercourse when it would not normally occur, and having intercourse without protection (either contraception or more probably protection from STDs). When a sexual history is taken, cofactors such as drugs should be ascertained and if drug use appears to be related to risk behaviours, then the practitioner should note this. The patient may have no conscious awareness of the part drug use may play in initiating sexual contact, or of its relationship with particularly risky behaviours. If this appears to be the case, then the practitioner should advise the patient of the risks involved where judgement is clouded. Unfortunately, alcohol and other drugs may be so closely associated with sexual contacts, both because of their disinhibiting action and because of the traditional relationship between sex and celebrations or bars and dances as places for making sexual contact, that awareness may not be translated into action.

It can be seen from these examples that there is considerable scope for the practitioner to engage in preventive health measures with patients in the area of sexual functioning. Generally raising the issue of preventive health care may also be a useful way of moving into the area of taking a sexual history. Of course, where a STD has been diagnosed, preventive education is mandatory (as described in the chapter on pre- and post-test counselling). However, preventive education in the area of sexual health should be seen as a part of general preventive health and medicine, and integrated into general patient and community primary prevention of health problems. In this context, a simple explanation of what can be prevented and why is a useful stimulus to motivating the patient to look after their own health and to promoting attendance for regular screening as appropriate.

References

1. Diamond, M. Sex and reproduction: conception and contraception. In Green, R. (ed.) *Human sexuality: a health practitioner's text* (2nd ed.) Baltimore: Williams & Wilkins, 1979: 58–80.
2. Brandt, A.M. *No magic bullet: a social history of veneral diseases in the United States since 1880.* New York: Oxford University Press, 1985.
3. Paavonen, J, Koutsky, L.A and Kiviat, N. Cervical neoplasms and other STD-related genital and anal neoplasms. In Holmes, K.K, Mårdh, P.A, Sparling, P.F and Wiesner, P.J. (eds) *Sexually transmitted diseases.* (2nd edn). New York: McGraw-Hill, 1990: 561–592.
4. Weström, L and Mårdh, P.A. Acute pelvic inflammatory disease. In Holmes, K.K, Mårdh, P.A, Sparling, P.F and Wiesner, P.J (eds) *Sexually transmitted diseases.* (2nd edn). New York: McGraw-Hill, 1990: 593–613.
5. Anderson, E.E. Early diagnosis of testicular carcinoma: self-examination of the testicle. *N Carolina Med J*, 1985: 46, 407–409.

CHAPTER 9

SEXUALITY AND CHRONIC ILLNESS

Although many chronic illnesses have an effect on sexuality, patients are notoriously reluctant to discuss the issue unless it is broached by the doctor. Studies of patient populations show that while many patients report sexual problems, few have mentioned them to their medical practitioner.[1] This may be a matter of reticence, or a preoccupation with more pressing concerns such as the possibility of a terminal illness.

It is therefore incumbent on the medical practitioner to introduce the question of the effect of illness on the patient's sexuality. Perhaps the best way to introduce the subject is to use a 'normalising' approach such as, 'Many people with your illness find they have some sexual problems. Have you noticed any difficulties since your illness began?'

Responses to this kind of advance vary enormously. A cheery couple in late middle age nodded happily to each other as the husband said, 'Oh, we're past all that, love'. A young married man who had had consultations with a broad range of health practitioners before reaching the pain clinic of a large public hospital was moved almost to tears. 'That's the very worst thing going wrong in my life and no-one's ever asked me about it before'. We have also been told to mind our own business.

The implication is plain. The issue needs to be broached in all cases of chronic illness but the physician needs to be sensitive to the fact that some patients will not have a problem and some will be simply unwilling to discuss any difficulties. The patient must, however, be given the choice.

Chronic illness can have both physical and psychological effects on sexuality. Box 9A lists some illnesses which frequently have physical effects on sexual performance and enjoyment.

Psychiatric disorders and sexuality

Analysis of the impact of psychiatric disorder on sexuality is difficult because of the confounding effects of medication. It is often hard to assess whether sexual dysfunction is a direct result of the psychiatric disorder or a side-effect of the long-term use of psychotropic drugs.

BOX 9A

Arthritis	Pain may make intercourse difficult. Involvement of the hip particularly may preclude intercourse.[5]
Asthma	Sexual arousal may be associated with attacks. A feedback loop may be set up with the patient becoming anxious and increasing the chances of an attack.[6]
Chronic benign pain	Reduction in intercourse frequency because of pain.[7]
Diabetes	While libido usually remains intact, about 50% of diabetic men suffer a degree of erectile dysfunction.[8]
Multiple sclerosis	Demyelination of neurones can affect erectile capacity, ejaculation, orgasm and movement.
Neurological damage	Many effects, depending on site, size and side of lesion.
Obstructive airways disease	Breathlessness detracts from sexual performance and enjoyment.[9]
Renal disease	Patients report loss of libido, anorgasmia and erectile dysfunction.[10]
Sleep apnoea	40% of male patients report erectile dysfunction. Moodiness disrupts relationships.[11]
Spinal injury	Depending on the level of injury, some or all of sexual sensation and function may be lost in both sexes.
Vascular disease	About half of male patients suffering from reduced blood circulation in the legs show erectile dysfunction. Anti-hypertensive drugs may also cause dysfunction.[13]

Loss of libido is one of the classic symptoms of severe depression. This will have an impact on the sexual relationship. It is worth remembering that depression features in many cases of chronic illness and that both monoamine oxidase inhibitors and tricyclic antidepressants have been found to reduce erectile and ejaculatory capacity.[2]

Some schizophrenic patients focus their delusions and hallucinations on sexual matters. More commonly, there is a reduction in sexual interest and fantasy. Nestos, Lehmann and Ban[3] studied hospitalised, medicated schizophrenic patients and found that many reported having no interest whatsoever in sexuality. A further confounding factor here is that many schizophrenic patients are socially withdrawn and hence unlikely to find a partner. Also, the policy of most psychiatric hospitals has been to discourage sexual activity between patients.

Substance abuse is usually deleterious to sexual well-being. Both acute and chronic alcohol over-use reduce the male's capacity for penile erection and the female's orgasmic capacity.

Barbiturates and stimulants can both affect sexual performance negatively. There have been some claims for an aphrodisiac effect from LSD, but the effect of the drug is unreliable. Similarly some people find that marijuana enhances sexual pleasure, specifically of orgasm.

Psychosocial effects of chronic illness

Changes in appearance either as a result of the illness or of treatment can be devastating to a person's sexual self-image. Hair loss resulting from chemotherapy, the surgical removal of a body part and so on can have a major impact. The patient feels unattractive and may assume that the partner will not welcome sexual advances.

Many chronically ill patients feel lethargic and simply cannot summon up the energy for intercourse.

Especially for patients recovering from stroke or myocardial infarct, there may be a fear that sexual activity will increase the risk of a second attack. The patient needs to be reassured that sexual activity, like any other form of moderate exercise, is actually beneficial to the cardiovascular system.

There is a need for careful inquiry about the effect of illness on the patient's relationship, as people vary tremendously in their response to illness. It may very well be a good idea to talk to the couple together (see chapter five) as the partners may not have communicated frankly and have quite erroneous impressions of what the other person is thinking and feeling.

Box 9B gives some common responses of patients and partners.

BOX 9B

Partnership reseponses to chronic illness

Responses from the patient

1. Concern about how the partner will feel about reduced sexual activity.
2. Anger, repressed or felt, that the partner is still healthy.
3. Guilt. The illness is a punishment and the patient deserves to lose the pleasures of sexuality.
4. Sexual frustration. This is especially so in a sexually-functioning patient who requires long periods of hospitalisation. Most hospitals pay little if any attention to the sexual needs of patients.
5. Use of the illness to break off sexual relations completely if the relationship was previously unsatisfactory.
6. Worries about possible infidelity by a frustrated partner.
7. Anxiety about possible sexual failure.
8. Concerns that changes in appearance may be unattractive.

Responses from the partner

1. Sexual frustration. This may lead to searching for another partner.
2. Anger because of deprivation.
3. Resentment of increased service demands.
4. Worry that sexual activity may damage the patient's health.
5. Use of the illness to break off sexual relations where they have previously been less than satisfactory.
6. Guilt that they themselves are not sick.
7. Distaste about changes in the patient's appearance.
8. An irrational belief that sexual relations may be contagious, especially seen when the patient has cancer.

Sexual rehabilitation

Dengrove[4] outlines some important factors in rehabilitation.

First, the quality of the sexual relationship before the illness is important. If the relationship had been a good one, one or both partners may feel deprived by the loss of a fulfilling part of life. If the relationship had been poor, one or both may use the illness as an excuse for ceasing sexual relationships altogether.

Secondly, the physical effects of the illness influence the extent to which rehabilitation is possible. As outlined in Box 9A many illnesses have direct effects on sexuality and libido. Others produce tiredness and a general lack of motivation, which includes sexual motivation.

Thirdly, the person's response to the illness in terms of its impact on sexual self-image is relevant. A woman who has had a radical mastectomy may feel very much less of a sexual being after the operation.

Various therapies may affect sexual function and sexual image. Medication may reduce erectile ability, reduce orgasmic capacity or lessen libido. Surgery such as mastectomy and hysterectomy may affect sexual self-image in women. Chemotherapy with its associated hair loss may make the patient feel unattractive or make the partner perceive the patient as sexually unattractive. It also tends to produce lethargy, which reduces the likelihood of the patient's engaging in sexual activity.

Lastly, the response of the patient and partner as a couple is relevant (see Box 9B).

These factors all need to be assessed, preferably with the patient and partner together. The couple may need the first three steps of the PLISSIT model — permission to discuss the issues, limited information and specific suggestions.

References

1. Schover, L.R and Jensen, S.B. *Sexuality and chronic illness. A comprehensive approach.* New York: The Guilford Press, 1988.
2. Dickes, R and Fleming, J.L. Sexuality in general medical practice. In R.C. Simons (ed.) *Understanding human behaviour in health and illness*, 3rd edn. Baltimore: Williams & Wilkins, 1985.
3. Nestoros, J.N, Lehmann, H.E and Ban, T.A. Sexual behaviour of the male schizophrenic: The impact of illness and medications. *Archives of Sexual Behaviour*, 1981: 10: 421–442.
4. Dengrove, E. Sexual responses to disease processes. *Journal of Sex Research*, 1968: 4, 257–264.
5. Ehrlich, G.E. Sexual problems and the arthritic patient. In: G.E. Ehrlich (ed.) *Total management of the arthritic patient*, Philadelphia: J.B. Lippincott, 1973.
6. Kaplan, R.M, Reis, A and Atkins, C.J. Behavioural issues in the management of chronic obstructive pulmonary disease. *Annals of Behavioural Medicine*, 1985: 7: 5–10.
7. Sjogren, K and Fugl-Meyer, A.R. Chronic back pain and sexuality. In *Rehab Med*, 1981: 3: 19–25.
8. Ellenberg, M. Impotence and diabetes mellitus: the neurological factor. *Ann of Intern Med*, 1971: 75: 213–219.
9. Hanson, E.I. Effects of chronic lung disease on life in general and on sexuality: perceptions of adult patients. *Heart and Lung*, 1982: 11: 435–431.

10. Abram, H.S. Sexual functioning in patients with chronic renal failure. *J Nerv Ment Dis*, 1975: 160; 220–226.
11. Singh, B. Sleep apnea: A psychiatric perspective. In N.A Saunders amd C.E. Sullivan (eds) *Sleep and breathing*. New York: Marcel Dekker, Inc., 1984.
12. Metz, P. Erectile dysfunction in men with occlusive arterial disease in the legs. *Dan Med Bull*, 1983: 30; 185–189.
13. Moss, H.B and Procci, W.R. Sexual dysfunction associated with oral antihypertensive medication: A critical survey of the literature. *General Hospital Psychiatry*, 1982: 4; 121–129.

CHAPTER 10

SEXUALITY AND DRUG-RELATED HISTORY

A number of drugs, both prescribed and social, may have an effect on sexual functioning. Such effects may be due to the direct action of the drug, an interaction between the drug and psychological factors, or in the case of prescribed drugs, a response to the illness for which the drug has been prescribed rather than the effect of the drug itself. It is not commonly appreciated that there may be an iatrogenic component to sexual dysfunctions. This may be through direct and indirect effects (for example through its effects on libido rather than on the physiology of sexual function) and appears more likely to affect male function than female function. The possibility of iatrogenic factors influencing or causing sexual dysfunction, as well as the fact that social drugs may also have the same effects, should make a history of medication and drug use mandatory when investigating sexual dysfunction. There are a number of ways drugs may affect sexual dysfunction.

Central nervous system depressants

Alcohol is the best known and probably most commonly implicated example of a CNS depressant with potential effects on sexual function. CNS depressants may act by reducing libido and causing sexual dysfunction secondary to this. However, the effect may be variable, for example a small amount of alcohol may increase libido but larger amounts decrease it. Alcohol in larger quantities has the classic acute effect of increasing desire but decreasing performance. Chronic alcohol use may not affect libido to the same extent as acute intoxication but is often associated with impotence. Chronic alcohol abuse may cause liver dysfunction which can then affect hormonal function, leading in extreme cases to feminisation in men or through damage to the peripheral nervous system interfere with the physical component of erection. Disturbance of the pituitary-gonadal axis from chronic alcohol consumption may also impair sexual response.

While CNS depressants may attenuate libido, and there is some suggestion that oral contraceptives in women may also reduce libido, in small doses anxiolytics may, like alcohol, initially increase libido but in larger doses reduce it.

Other drugs

Opioids: Opioids may have a complex effect on sexual function. In addition to their effect on CNS function, they will have a sedative effect and will increase prolactin release which will in turn inhibit sexual function.

Antihypertensives: Some antihypertensives (for example, thiazide diuretics) have been implicated in erectile dysfunction and may also interfere with ejaculation (adrenergic neuron blockers). Some such as methyldopa and clonidine have their influence by acting as CNS depressants. Beta blockers have only minor effects on sexual function. Drugs which interfere with the sympathetic nervous system may cause failure of ejaculation and secondarily, via psychological mechanisms, sexual dysfunction.

Anticholinergic agents: Many drugs have anticholinergic properties, and thus may have an effect on sexual function by interfering with erection which is dependent on sacral para-sympathetic function. Tricyclic antidepressants and some of the classical antipsychotic agents such as chlorpromazine and thioridazine may have this effect. Classical antihistamine agents such as anti-motion sickness preparations may also affect sexual function in the same way as well as through their sedating effects.

Agents which increase prolactin secretion: Such agents decrease the release of gonadotrophins from the pituitary and thus secondarily gonadal hormone release. This ultimately is associated with decreased libido and secondary sexual dysfunction. The commonest mechanism for increasing prolactin is by blockade of dopamine receptors in the hypothalamus by drugs such as antipsychotics and also the antiemetic metoclopramide.

There are a number of other drugs which have been associated with sexual dysfunction, although the mechanisms for their effect are not necessarily understood. There is some suggestion from large controlled trials of the treatment of hypertension that thiazide diuretics may increase the incidence of erectile dysfunction, and that overdose of levodopa in Parkinsonian men has resulted in sexual disinhibition, which suggests that dopamine is involved as a neurotransmitter in mediating sexual response. Other drugs which have been reported to affect sexual functioning include some anti-migraine preparations, and H2 blockers such as cimetidine.

Hormones

***Anti-androgens*:** In the male, anti-androgens will decrease sexual functioning. They operate by reducing libido and thus causing secondary erectile dysfunction. Such drugs (progesterone analogues) may be given to sexual offenders to reduce libido. In general, any agent which decreases testicular function (and thus the production of testosterone), such as cytotoxic agents for treatment of malignancies, will have an effect on sexual function. Provision of androgens to normal males will have no physical effect, although in androgen deficient men, androgen supplementation will increase libido. Similarly, oestrogens in normal women will have no effect on sexual functioning, although in post-menopausal women may increase vaginal lubrication and thus have a secondary effect on sexual function by making intercourse less painful.

Social drugs

Sexual function may be affected by social drugs, the most common of which is alcohol. However, illicit opioid users will also experience the effects noted above for opioids. The more widespread use of illicit amphetamines also deserves consideration. There have been reports that there is a heightening of sexual interest when coming down from some amphetamines (particularly methamphetamines) and other amphetamine users have reported they enhance sexual experience. However, there has been little systematic work on this class of agents from the sexual direction.

The literature on cannabis provides conflicting data on many aspects of its use. However, one study does suggest that there may be a higher incidence of erectile dysfunction and decrease in sperm production. Volatile nitrites, inhaled by some homosexual men to heighten the experience of orgasm, do not appear to alter sexual function.

The role of social drugs should be considered not only in relation to their direct effects on sexual function, but in relation to their indirect effects in accompanying sexual behaviour which may be unsafe (in terms of STD and HIV transmission) and disinhibiting individuals who may have sexual relationships or engage in sexual acts they may otherwise not take part in. Thus, any STD history should also be accompanied by a history of the pharmacological climate of the risk behaviours.

Clinical considerations

Clinically, the commonest presentation of sexual dysfunction will be psychogenic. This will include people who are also on medication and have no direct effects of their drugs on sexual functioning. However, it is important for the practitioner to exclude pharmacological factors which may either primarily or secondarily affect sexual functioning, and to consider both prescribed and socially used agents. Drugs may affect different aspects of sexual functioning, and the health practitioner should be aware of the different ways in which particular agents may impact on sexual response. There may also be a spurious association of drugs and sexual functioning secondary to the illness being treated, (see particularly the previous chapter on the effect of chronic illness on sexuality) rather than a cause and effect relationship. In relation to general treatment, it should also be noted that if an agent does affect sexual functioning, then this will often affect compliance with the drug regimen.

In conclusion, while the health practitioner is likely to find that the great majority of cases of sexual dysfunction are psychogenic, they should also maintain a high index of suspicion for possible iatrogenic contributions to sexual dysfunction, and this index of suspicion should extend to socially used drugs. It is important to exclude pharmacological and physical factors when considering the differential diagnoses for sexual dysfunctions and this should include taking a drug use history during the sexual history.

CHAPTER 11

PRE-TEST AND POST-TEST COUNSELLING

The issue of appropriate pre-and post-test screening and counselling has a number of implications for correct counselling and management. For major problems such as HIV (and to a lesser extent, genital herpes) which at present can be controlled but not cured, adequate preparation serves both a preventive role in educating the patient to avoid further transmitting the infection, and prepares for and mitigates the major psychosocial morbidity which may arise from receiving a positive result. In some states, adequate pre- and post test counselling for HIV is mandatory by law. Thus for reasons of both law and good practice as well as preventive health care, pre- and post-test counselling is an important part of clinical practice for the management of viral STDs.

Pre-test counselling for HIV screening

Screening for antibodies to the human immunodeficiency virus (HIV) has become a reasonably common procedure since the test became available in April 1985. The more recent awareness that knowledge of HIV antibody status (or knowledge of status as a person with herpes) may be detrimental to an individual's mental health has, however, developed more slowly, although it is now well recognised[12] (Goldmeier and colleagues, 1988 for herpes; Ross and Rosser, 1988 for HIV infection). In about one third of cases the general practitioner is the point of testing, but little attention has been given to the practicalities of pretest counselling or the medical and ethical considerations attendant on testing.

Screening versus diagnostic testing

A distinction must be made between diagnostic testing and screening, since the ethical considerations are somewhat different. Further, diagnostic testing will be applicable to HIV and herpes, while screening is applicable to HIV. Screening describes the process of testing to provide early detection and treatment of a condition. In the case of HIV, there is no cure (although experimental trials of drugs are ongoing) and it is arguable that there is much benefit to the patient to know their HIV serostatus. In some cases there may be positive disadvantages. It has been argued that if there is nothing the practitioner can do to treat the seropositive individual, and the patient's knowledge of their seropositive status may lead to adverse psychological sequelae, then the principle *primum non nocere* (above all, do no harm) should apply, and the test be avoided. However, the fact that drugs such as azidothymidine (for HIV) and acyclovir (for herpes) can successfully treat (although not cure) these infections now weights the considerations in favour of knowing one's HIV serostatus.

Knowledge of viral STD infection, on the other hand, may lead the individual to modify lifestyle factors to prevent viral transmission. However, there have also been cases reported where the opposite has occurred, and individuals have set out to infect others, either deliberately or unconsciously, in their anger at finding themselves seropositive.[3] The general practitioner must therefore make a decision as to whether HIV antibody screening is indicated for the individual patient in terms of its probable sequelae. On the other hand, such reactions also make one of the strongest cases for adequate pre- and post-test counselling.

Diagnostic testing, on the other hand, is easier to justify than screening because in most cases it conveys an advantage in permitting differential diagnosis (which may include HIV infection, or herpes infection) to proceed. Further, with the possibility of treatment of both herpes and HIV infections, it is easier to justify. Nevertheless, the practitioner must still be aware of the potential psychosocial consequences and make a decision on whether the patient should be given pretest counselling and how they should be informed of the results. We present here a guide to how HIV counselling (and to a lesser extent herpes counselling) should proceed in health practice, and the considerations underlying this model. These are arranged in the suggested order of counselling and under major areas it is necessary to cover. While we refer to HIV as the exemplar because it is the most extreme situation, the arguments also apply (although usually with a lesser level of stigma and with a non-fatal outcome) for genital herpes simplex infection. Where herpes differs, this is noted. Otherwise, what is described for HIV will also apply although without quite the same degree of emotional trauma overall, for herpes.

Reasons for test: Most patients will present specifically requesting the HIV test. It is important to ascertain whether testing is necessary, since there has been extensive media coverage both nationally and internationally (most recently for AIDS; in the early 1980s for herpes) which has led to many misconceptions and, in some cases, hysteria. Further, some individuals may present in the absence of any risk. There are two other important reasons in ascertaining a need for testing:

1. The practitioner has an obligation in terms of primary prevention to provide information that ensures that patients do not transmit the virus if they are infected (and do not acquire STD viral infection if they are uninfected).
2. If individuals are AIDS or STD phobic,[4] testing may reinforce their irrational disease conviction.

The first step is thus to determine whether the test is appropriate and whether patients may have been exposed to infection.

Risk-taking behaviours: It is important not to phrase the query on risks of infection in terms of 'risk groups'. While epidemiologically certain groups currently show a greater prevalence of HIV or herpes infection, the statistical inference from a population to an individual is not valid, and may lead both to advising testing where inappropriate and not testing where appropriate. Some individuals may, for example, be homosexual but at no risk by virtue of their specific sexual practices.[5] Others may consider themselves heterosexual but nevertheless engage in same-sex practices: Kinsey, Pomeroy and Martin[6] found that 37% of men had had at least one homosexual encounter to orgasm between the ages of 16 and 65 years. Still others may be unaware of their partner's lifestyle or past experience which in turn has placed them at risk. Patients should initially be asked what specific behaviours or practices have put them at risk of viral infection. These practices include:

- Genital sexual intercourse (anal or vaginal) with multiple partners
- Sharing of needles during intravenous drug use
- Transfusion of blood or blood products up to April 1985
- Needlestick injury or mucocutaneous exposure to HIV seropositive (or possibly seropositive) individual
- Oral sexual intercourse (at present a theoretical risk)
- Artificial insemination by donor with untested semen
- In pediatric cases, mother virus seropositive pre-or perinatally

While genital or oral sexual intercourse with condoms markedly reduces risk of infection, cases have been reported where condoms did not provide protection against HIV infection.[7] Where condoms are inappropriately used or of inferior quality, the risk of infection may increase by a factor of ten.[7]

Reactions to test: Most individuals request the HIV antibody test with the assumption that they will be seronegative. Usually they will not have thought about the possibility of a positive result. It is imperative to ask what their reaction would be if the test proved to be positive. Their response to this question is one of the best indicators of their actual post seropositive reaction, and serves to both alert the patient to the possibility of negative sequelae, and to introduce them to the fact that there may be negative and harmful consequences arising from a screening test. Response to this question should also alert the practitioner to both potential psychological difficulties if the result proves positive, and to factors which may contraindicate the test. Essentially, the clinical dictum is that if the patient could not take a positive result, they should not take the test.

Individuals who indicate that they would hit out sexually following a positive result should also be advised against being tested. If the patient could, in the clinician's opinion, cope with a positive result, coping mechanisms should next be investigated.

Coping mechanisms: It is important to gain some insight into the patient's previous mechanisms of coping with stress, as this will provide one of the best indicators of how the individual will cope with a positive test result. Answers to the questions, 'What major stresses have you had in your life to date? How did (or would) you cope with them?' alert the practitioner to the potential need for support following a confirmed test result, to possible psychological decompensation, suicide attempt, refuge in alcohol or other drugs, or denial. If the practitioner believes the patient's life may be at risk following advice of a positive result, or that the life of a third party may be at risk, they should again give very serious consideration to not carrying out the test or, if the test is carried out, to providing appropriate support for the patient.

Concurrent stressors affecting the patient should also be investigated. Clinical experience has demonstrated that a positive HIV antibody or herpes test result may exacerbate any current difficulty in functioning. Specifically, major crises in the last 12 months prior to testing should be investigated and where present and unresolved, testing is usually contraindicated.

Social supports: One of the best predictors of longer term mental health is the degree of social support available to the individual. In the case that the patient is acceptable for testing so far, it is important for the practitioner to ascertain what social supports are available to the patient and any possible complications which may arise from the need to confide in inappropriate individuals. Choice of inappropriate support may lead to discrimination and further distress. Examples of this include confiding in individuals who then broadcast the fact that the patient 'has AIDS' or 'has herpes', and consequent discrimination in or eviction from accommodation, or harrassment at or dismissal from employment. Confiding in inappropriate individuals may also lead to the partial or complete loss of social supports at the time when the individual is most in need of them, with potentially serious consequences for mental health. The clinician may need to give consideration to providing such support or referral to agencies which provide support.

Mental history: If responses to questions relating to how the patient would cope with a positive test result, coping with previous stresses, and social supports reveal evidence that the patient may be at risk physically or psychologically from a positive result, then further details should be sought. Such details will include previous history of mental illness, suicidal ideation or suicide attempts, treatment for anxiety or depression, psychotherapy, or psychosis. Any history of severe depresion with suicidal ideation, or of psychosis, will raise serious questions as to the advisability of screening. If the test is indicated in differential diagnosis and a positive result is found, it is advisable to have adequate psychological follow-up and a high index of suspicion for changes in psychological state.

Provision of education: In the absence of a cure or vaccine for HIV or herpes infection in the foreseeable future, there is an absolute obligation for the health practitioner to provide education and to enhance the patient's primary preventive techniques. In addition to questions the patient may have raised in the course of the consultation, the following information must be provided as an absolute minimum:

- A positive HIV antibody test or herpes diagnostic test result indicates that the individual has been infected, is currently infected, and is likely to remain infectious for life.

- A person who is HIV antibody positive or herpes positive is infectious to others, but only under certain circumstances where there is transfer of body fluids (particularly blood, semen, and vaginal secretions).
- The individual has an obligation not to infect others if infected, and if uninfected should take all possible steps to remain that way. This includes avoidance of unsafe sex in which transfer of body fluids may occur, and not sharing needles during intravenous drug use. Reduction of sexual partners to a minimum and use of condoms to reduce risk of infection should be advised.

This information should be provided **before** testing, and certainly prior to the provision of the test result. Information provided at the same time as the test result is usually not remembered in the euphoria of a negative result or lost in the shock of a positive result.

Informed consent: The fact that HIV screening may have negative consequences for the individual should be discussed with the patient for consent to be fully informed. The following areas must be covered:

- There is no cure currently available (other than for treatment of opportunistic infections). Those treatments available can reduce progression of disease. If there is a positive result this **may** in some cases reduce transmission from the infected person but this is not universal. There is thus advantage to others, but not necessarily the individual, in taking the test
- The result of a positive test may lead to psychological decompensation (breakdown or inability to cope), depression and anxiety
- The person must be made aware of the relevant state laws relating to notification and penalties associated with transmission of the virus
- The patient must be made aware of the potential infringement of rights (loss of housing, employment) arising from potential breaches of confidentiality, and the potential disadvantages of divulging positive HIV antibody status to third parties
- Life insurance will not be available to individuals who are HIV antibody positive.

In providing information on the negative aspects of testing, it becomes clear that the test at this point in time does not offer a great deal to the individual, although there are considerable benefits to society in terms of provision of epidemiological information on which to base drug trials and monitor the effectiveness of prevention programmes.

As with other medical procedures, however, consent is not held to be informed if potential disadvantages are not discussed. Although to date there have not been any cases to provide guidelines, there are a number of potential medicolegal issues involved in HIV antibody testing, with informed consent and the basis of the clinical decision to carry out testing, being the two most prominent ones.

Preventive counselling

In the absence of a cure, the health practitioner has an obligation to encourage primary prevention in those who present, whether specifically for the HIV antibody test and herpes diagnostic test or those whose lifestyle or behaviour put them at risk of infection. It must be noted that testing is not essential to prevention, for if all individuals avoided behaviours which put them at risk of HIV infection, the spread of this epidemic would cease.

Central to the prevention of the virus's spread is advice on limiting sexual contacts to one or only a few regular partners without outside contacts or, if this is not possible, avoidance of sexual practices which may transfer body fluids (anal or vaginal intercourse, and possibly oral intercourse) or appropriate condom use.

Advice on condom use needs to be specific and behaviourally oriented. Research into heterosexual use of condoms shows that when used properly, failure rate is less than 3/100 woman years, although in general usage it may rise to 10/100 woman years.[9]

For intravenous drug users, it is important to provide advice on the necessity of not sharing needles and information on where to obtain sterile equipment if sharing is not avoidable.

Once individuals are aware of how HIV or herpes are transmitted, they can play an active part in reducing infection. Intravenous drug users have been identified as a particularly difficult group to educate. Education of individual patients may well be a key element in informing the wider subculture through encouraging patients to pass relevant information on informally to fellow users.

Efficacy of testing

The assumption is frequently made that testing for HIV will encourage individuals to prevent or avoid viral transmission. The evidence on this is ambiguous, with one study showing that while individuals who are seropositive reduce partner numbers by up to 50%, seronegative individuals show little reduction. On the other hand, further studies have showed that individuals who did not know their antibody status after testing showed no reduction in partner numbers. When the effects of counselling alone, testing alone, testing plus counselling, and no intervention were compared on AIDS prophylactic behaviours in homosexual men, it was found that counselling and testing were more effective than testing only, which in turn was more effective than counselling alone, which had more effect than no intervention.[10] It would seem reasonable to conclude that counselling does enhance the effect of testing, and that testing may have benefits in terms of reduction of viral spread. However, the role of the health practitioner is to identify those individuals for whom testing would be advantageous, and to refer on for a further opinion those for whom a positive test result would lead to harm or to increased viral transmission. For those who may be harmed by a positive test result, but for whom the medical practitioner believes the test to be appropriate on balance, more intensive follow-up and support is recommended.

Other sexually transmitted diseases

If a patient is judged to be at risk of HIV infection through sexual contact or genital herpes infection, then they will also be at risk from other sexually transmitted diseases (STDs). It is important for the practitioner to be aware of this and to concurrently test for other diseases. This should include syphilis serology, hepatitis B serology, and swabbing appropriate sites (including vagina, urethra, rectum and mouth) for gonorrhoea and chlamydia. If the practitioner does not feel competent to carry out full venereological examination, referral should be made to a local STD clinic. It is important not to forget that AIDS is primarily a STD and that while patients may not be infected with HIV, they may carry other STDS which require treatment. The high proportion of STDs which are asymptomatic reinforces the importance of such concurrent screening.

Recording HIV tests and results

The possibility of discrimination (real or imagined) against patients, if their results were to be disclosed to others, has led to considerable concern about confidentiality. This may include concern about results being communicated to reception staff or to members of the patient's family or spouse (particularly where family members are seen by the same practitioner or at the same practice). Reassurance of confidentiality is therefore appropriate. Common practices to ensure confidentiality may include providing a code (or alias) on specimens or request forms, and keeping a private or locked register of such codes or aliases. Recording of results on patient files has not provided adequate protection of confidentiality in some hospital settings[11] and may be similarly inadequate in private settings or where many personnel have access to patient files. These issues do need to be considered and patients may request specific reassurance on matters of confidentiality which we are accustomed to take for granted.

Post-test counselling for HIV screening

Post-test counselling is complementary to pre-test counselling, and the counselling described here is that which will follow such pre-test counselling. Again, we use HIV infection as the exemplar but find this to be equally applicable to genital herpes infection (although there is usually less trauma involved). It must be emphasised that results should not be given over the telephone (regardless of whether they are positive or negative), and that at the time of the test an appointment should be made to return for the test results. When the practitioner sees the patient, they will have in front of them the notes of the pre-test counselling and will proceed on the basis of these and of the test results. Essentially, results will be either positive or negative (for HIV, positive on a screening test such as ELISA and positive on a confirmatory test such as western blot). Unconfirmed positives should not be provided given the possibility, albeit very small, of false positives. In the rare case of indeterminate results, the result should be treated as positive until proven otherwise. Post-test counselling can conveniently be divided into counselling of people with positive or negative results.

Post-test counselling for negative results

Such counselling, provided that pre-test counselling has been adequately carried out, need not be time-consuming. It has to take into account that a negative result may be taken as a 'license to fly' and that the message that it takes only one incident of unsafe behaviour to infect the person must be the first and foremost one.

The second purpose of post-test counselling for negative results is to reiterate the information on how the virus is transmitted. Unless there has been any indication of failure to grasp the information in the pre-test counselling session, this can be in the form of briefly going over what is 'safe' in the way of sex (no penetrative sex) or 'safer' (penetrative sex using a condom). In the case of genital herpes, this will include specific instructions on the risk of transmission even when vesicles or ulceration are not present. In the case of injecting drugs, unused injecting equipment is 'safe' from the point of HIV transmission: cleaning with bleach, disinfectant or alcohol (two pre-rinses, two rinses in bleach, two cleaning rinses) is 'safer'. It is important to make clear the difference between 'safe' and 'safer'. 'Safe' means that there is no chance of transmitting HIV or herpes. 'Safer' means that the chance is reduced but that accidents (such as condom breakage, improper application, or inadequate cleaning of injecting equipment) can still not be ruled out.

If the patient has had repeated tests, it may be advisable to make time to do a fuller assessment. This can be appropriate in two situations. First, if risk behaviour continues and the patient seems to regard a negative test as licensing further unsafe behaviour (or even as confirming or reinforcing that previous unsafe behaviour carries no risk), then the situation needs to be addressed clearly.

Second, patients may present for repeated testing in the absence of reported risk behaviours. If one is fairly certain that the patient is reporting risk behaviours accurately, then this raises the possibility of abnormal behaviour (see the previous chapter on diagnosis and counselling for STDs) which should be addressed. Finally, the post-test counselling session provides an opportunity for the patient to clarify any matters which might have been raised and not completely understood or answered in the pre-test counselling session, or which have arisen since and require clarification.

Post-test counselling for positive results

This presents one of the most difficult situations for both practitioner and patient. It may have ramifications in clinical and psychological terms far beyond the initial fact of HIV or genital herpes infection, and the practitioner will probably have to deal at least with the immediate manifestations of these. On the other hand, if the pre-test counselling has been carried out, giving a positive result will be resting on a solid foundation. The practitioner will already know what chance the patient thinks they have of being infected, and how the patient thinks they would deal with a positive result, as well as having some idea of previous psychological difficulties (if any). The pre-test counselling has been designed to make post-test counselling as well-informed and appropriate as possible, and has set the stage in an interpersonal sense for practitioner and patient to have some sort of clinical relationship.

Advising a patient of results: Because of the trauma associated with positive results, adequate time (a minimum of half an hour, preferably more) should be allocated. Positive results should **not** be given on the telephone or on a walk in, walk out basis. Such a method of telling patients often reinforces the idea that they are 'lepers' and makes it difficult if not impossible for the practitioner to make an assessment of the patient's mental state or need for further support or services. If the result is not expected by the patient, then the news is likely to be even more psychologically traumatising.

Does the patient want to know?: First ascertain that the patient has come for the test result. In rare cases, the patient may have decided that they don't want to know, and this should be respected. They may also have come to talk further about the issue before deciding to ask for their result.

Breaking the news: There is no easy way to break the news, and this section concentrates on the situation of HIV infection. However, the responses to news of herpes infection and counselling will follow the same pattern. If the practitioner prevaricates, or prefaces the news with a statement about how HIV infection doesn't necessarily lead to AIDS, they have already given the news, and in addition the information that the practitioner has trouble coping with it. The result is to make the patient feel that if the practitioner has trouble coping with it, how can the patient be expected to manage?

The issue of giving positive HIV results has been dealt with in some detail by Green and McCreaner,[12] and readers wanting to look at scenarios and role-plays of post-test counselling should refer to this book. Essentially, Green and McCreaner state that it is best to tell the patient straightforwardly, without evasion or qualification, what the results are. Any evasion or qualification may confuse the patient to the point where they are unsure exactly what the results are. Thus the post-test counselling **starts** with the facts (that the test result is positive, and that the patient has been infected with HIV, the virus which may cause AIDS).

Focusing on the response: At this point, there is a tendency for the practitioner to launch into explanations or qualifications. Don't. First, the patient may be in a state of shock and will not be able to take in much of what you are saying. Second, we are doing post-test counselling for the benefit of the patient's psychological state as much as for information. The next step is to focus on the patient's response by making a statement in the form of a question such as 'You seem quite surprised: did you expect this?' or 'This seems to come as a real shock to you?', or even 'I guess that this raised a lot of new issues for you'. These questions give the patient the opportunity to tell one **what** issues are immediate and uppermost in their mind, and what order they want to cope with things in. This gives the practitioner the clue as to where to proceed on the **patient's** agenda.

Coping with the news: The reactions of people to the news will vary considerably. Responses will range from relief to have what was suspected confirmed, through to denial or inability to handle the information. It is important to let the patient describe their response and set the direction of the consultation. Green and McCreaner report that responses tend to fall into three main categories.

First, there may be statements such as comments of confirmation or denial of the possibility. The practitioner should indicate that they are listening and encourage the patient to go on. *Second*, there may be reactions such as silence or tears. There is a temptation to fill in difficult moments with talk. Avoid this: instead, if there is silence, ask the patient to verbalise their thoughts (there may be many things going through their minds) as this will help the practitioner to determine what the central problems are. If the patient cries, again resist the temptation to distract or talk yourself. Seek clarification when appropriate by asking a question such as 'What do you find most upsetting about the result?'.

The *third* response is a question. This may range from a factual question to a rhetorical one such as 'How will I tell ...?'. These latter questions which cover areas about what the patient will do, and how they will organise their existence around their HIV serostatus (or herpes infection), are not actually asking the practitioner for an answer. Green and McCreaner suggest that they are an invitation to discuss the issue from a number of different angles. Reflecting back the question ('You're worried about how X will react?' or 'How do you think that will affect them?') is probably the best way of starting into the discussion.

Most common mistakes: On talking with patients about how they would prefer to be told, and what went wrong, a number of common mistakes emerge. The most common is information overload. The patient is often sitting in a state of shock or contemplation and the session is filled with the practitioner talking. In a state of anxiety, the patient will either take little in, or worse, get the information muddled or wrong because they are only partially attending. Until you cope with the psychological reaction, it is pointless to give a lecture on the meaning of the result.

A second common mistake is not to provide the patient with the time and opportunity to come to terms with the information at their own pace. It is important to **follow up** the patient because after the interview they will certainly have many questions which they want to ask, or even just an opportunity to talk about the situation later in a more prepared fashion. The worst thing the practitioner can do is to give the result and then leave the patient to their own devices. At a minimum, a further appointment should be made, and either an after-hours number given with the invitation to call when the patient needs reassurance or information, or the number of an AIDS Hotline or information service given. Don't leave the patient without a lifeline.

The third common mistake is to be too technical. Most patients will not have degrees in medical science, so tailor your provision of information to their level. It is not uncommon to have patients complain that they didn't understand a word of what they were told by a practitioner because it was so technical. Even concepts such as latency, defence systems and germs may be too much for some patients. The message is simple, so keep it that way, and encourage questions so that patients can learn more if they want to, and so that you can get an idea of what they really understand.

Discussing the issues: There will be a number of issues raised by the patient which need to be discussed. These will include several mandatory pieces of information. First, it must be made clear that in the case of HIV infection, being infected does not mean that the patient will necessarily go on to fully developed AIDS, and that HIV infection is not the same thing. Of course, if the patient shows signs or symptoms of AIDS, it would not be appropriate to raise this issue. Second, the issue of who should be told must be raised. It is not uncommon for patients to be sufficiently distraught as to tell people who on reflection are inappropriate, and this may often lead to the information being widely and indiscriminately spread. Alternatively, it may also lead to discrimination and rejection. Because the patient will want to confide in and receive support from significant others, this issue should be raised and social support mechanisms assessed.

At this stage, the practitioner is making an assessment as to whether the psychological response is appropriate or whether there may be additional issues arising. If patients have a history of depression, suicide attempts, or have indicated in pre-test counselling that this is something they have considered, referral for psychiatric assessment and until this occurs, close monitoring, is mandatory. In cases such as this it may be wise to give the patient the practitioner's after hours number or to advise the locum or covering practitioner of the situation.

One of the central issues in the discussion (which may cover more than one session) is coping with the diagnosis. When the patient raises such issues, rather than focussing on the inability to cope, try to make a list of the problems foreseen. Then go down the list and take the problem which appears to be most amenable to solution, and elicit from the patient the possibilities for managing the issue. In the first session, if there is time, try to cover only one or two and leave others until later sessions if possible to avoid overload.

Remember that if the patient is shocked by the test result, they will tend to see things fairly negatively and thus attempting to force concentration on issues of coping (particularly when it may take some time for the news to sink in) is inappropriate. These matters should be dealt with as raised by the patient (possibly with some gentle encouragement) and not laid on them when they may be unable to cope with them.

Finally, there is one piece of good news that can be given to most patients (unless they present with signs or symptoms of AIDS). There is no reason at all that a person with HIV or genital herpes infection cannot lead a normal life and have a reasonable life expectancy after infection. This should be emphasised, with the patient being encouraged to see the question as being one of continuing their life rather than seeing it as ending.

Even in the most difficult situation, don't take all hope away from the patient.

Concluding the session: Reassurance of the fact that the practitioner will not abandon the patient, and confirmation of one's concern and willingness to assist are an important aspect of the end of the consultation. While this may be taken for granted by the clinician, there are enough stories, both true and apocryphal, of rejection of patients by practitioners and sufficient evidence of stigmatisation of HIV- and herpes-infected people, to make this mandatory. Patients have described in graphic terms the trauma of receiving a positive result from an HIV test[13] or genital herpes test[14] and thus it is also mandatory to make a follow-up appointment at a mutually agreed time in the next few days to reassess the patient's mental state and coping strategies, and to provide support or referral as appropriate.

Issues for a later session: Because AIDS is a high-profile epidemic (as herpes was in the early 1980s), unlike other infections, patients may be quite well informed through the media and frequently confronted with increasingly pessimistic morbidity and mortality statistics. While health practitioners are often asked for precise information on the likelihood and timing of disease progression in the case of HIV, such information is unlikely to be of benefit to the patient and may encourage a sense of fatalism or despair. Where patients are aware of such statistics, it is important not to remove all hope. There is a great deal of variation in statistics on progression rates, and thus provision of specific statistics may not enhance the reputation of the clinician for reliability of information should estimates change (as they frequently will in the light of more recent studies).

There are a number of other issues which should be addressed at a subsequent session. These include provision of information about the disease, when the patient is able to take it in, discussion of the implications of the disease (on relationships, on sexual response, on having children, on life insurance, on work, on stigmatisation, on health care and vaccinations, and on donation of body tissue (including blood).

The patient with HIV infection should be warned of any symptoms which may indicate opportunistic infection, and encouraged to seek a medical opinion if these occur. However, it is important to make this matter of fact and simple, or one is only encouraging hypochondriasis or excessive preoccupation with bodily symptoms.

One of the important concerns of people with HIV infection is an apparent lack of control over disease progression (and with herpes, control over disease expression). This must be addressed for both physical and psychological reasons.[15] From the physical point of view, there are a number of drugs and drug trials available, and they should be discussed with the patient. Disease progression or expression can probably be influenced by sensible diet, exercise, and looking after oneself. Reduction of stress and adequate relaxation are also factors which may slow progression of disease, particularly in the case of herpes. Thus, there are a number of steps that the patient can take to maintain their health and possibly to slow disease progression or expression.

There are also a number of more traditional complementary therapies which should not be discouraged if they do no harm. Giving some control back to the patient to maintain hope and to assist in maintaining health can have positive effects on both physical and mental health.

If patients are going to become anxious, depressed or suicidal it is not uncommon for this to occur in the first days or weeks following a positive result. If this is explained to the patient, and the possibility of distress acknowledged, it makes it easier for the patient to make contact before an extreme situation develops. At the psychological level, psychological control can be encouraged by discussing with the patient the things which are likely to trigger anxiety or depression, and suggesting that they should try to avoid such situations if possible. Awareness of the onset of depression should also be encouraged, and the patient encouraged to seek help if there are changes to sleep patterns, appetite, or increasing helplessness or hopelessness. Most depressive illnesses and anxiety states can be easily treated, and there is no reason why people should be condemned to misery or dis-ease where amelioration is available. Given the possibility of psychological dis-ease in people with HIV infection, it should be made clear that this is not something that has to be borne but that treatment for this should be sought in the same way as physical symptoms should be recognised and attended to.

Referral: If the practitioner is not prepared or competent to care for the patient themselves, they will need to be referred to a specialist or clinic for immunological work-up. The patient may see this as a rejection because of their HIV or genital herpes status, so it is important to make it clear that this is for specialist attention and not because the practitioner can't cope with an HIV seropositive or herpes infected patient. Unfortunately, nearly one quarter of medical practitioners recently surveyed in Australia said they would not be prepared to treat an HIV seropositive patient, so the fears of the patient may be realistic.

Where there are psychological sequelae or previous or concurrent psychological disturbance, psychiatric referral, or referral to a clinic with psychological services, should also occur unless the practitioner is comfortable and competent in dealing with psychological illness or maladjustment.

In summary, post-test counselling, if the patient is HIV seropositive or has genital herpes, may appear to be one of the most difficult consultations for both practitioner and patient. However, there are a number of common issues which arise and the session usually follows a distinct form. If the practitioner bears this in mind and follows these guide-lines, much of the discomfort and difficulty should be avoided and the session will benefit the patient and their response to their infection. The key to appropriate post-test counselling is to attend to the psychological issues before attending to the informational ones, and take the cues from the patient as to the amount of time that will need to be devoted to each.

Conclusion

These guide-lines outline the role of the general practitioner (and other medical specialists who may become involved in HIV or herpes testing) in making a clinical judgement on the appropriateness of testing, the conduct of pre- and post-test counselling, and some of the medical, psychosocial and medicolegal issues involved. It is important to note that HIV testing may have both positive and negative outcomes in terms of both the individual and the spread of the disease, and there is an obligation to assess each applicant for testing to determine whether the test is appropriate. In the case of a screening test, for HIV antibodies, where there is no treatment if the test does prove positive, and real harm may result from the patient's knowledge of their infection, adequate assessment in order to 'do no harm' is an important aspect of the exercise of clinical judgement.

The role of the health practitioner is central in dealing with HIV and genital herpes infection. The general practitioner will frequently be the first point of contact for the anxious and for those wanting a test for evidence of HIV infection, and can play a major and most productive part in preventive medicine. In the support and routine medical care of those who are infected, the general practitioner will again play one of the most important roles in the management of HIV infection and AIDS and herpes, as well as many other sexually transmissible diseases.

References

1. Goldmeier, D, Johnson, A, Byrne, M and Barton, S. Psychosocial implications of recurrent genital herpes simplex virus infection. *Genitourinary Medicine*, 1988: 64, 327–330.

2. Ross, M.W and Rosser, B.R.S. Counselling issues in AIDS-related syndroimes: a review. *Patient Education and Counselling*, 1988: 11, 17–28.
3. Spencer, J and Grey, J. AIDS: two case histories. *Aust Fam Physician*, 1986: 15(1), 36–38.
4. Ross, M.W. AIDS phobias: a report of four cases. *Psychopathology* 1988: 21; 26–30.
5. Ross, M.W. Social and behavioral aspects of male homosexual behavior. In: Coney, T.G and Ward, T.T. (eds) *AIDS and other medical problems in the male homosexual*. Philadelphia: W.B. Saunders, 1986.
6. Kinsey, A.C, Pomeroy, W.B and Martin, C.E. *Sexual behaviour in the human male*. Philadelphia: W.B. Saunders, 1948.
7. Fischl, M.A, Dickinson, G.M, Scott, G.B, Klimas, N, Fletcher, M.A and Parks, W. Evaluation of heterosexual partners, children and household contacts of adults with AIDS. *Journal of the American Medical Association*, 1987: 257; 640–644.
8. Bell, J. The thin latex line against disease. *New Scientist*, 1987: 1549, 58.
9. Dunn, K and Leeton, J. *Birth control*. Melbourne: Pitman, 1982.
10. Ross, M.W. The relationship of combinations of AIDS counselling and testing to safer sex and condom use in homosexual men. *Community Health Studies*, 1988: 12, 322–327.
11. Cohen, M.A and Weisman, H.W. A biopsychosocial approach to AIDS. *Psychosomatics*, 1986: 27; 245–255.
12. Green, J and McCreaner, A. Post-test counselling. In: Green, J and McCreaner, A. (eds) *Counselling in HIV infection and AIDS*. Oxford: Blackwell, 1989: 28–68.
13. Richards, T. Don't tell me on a friday. *Br Med J*, 1986: 292; 943–945.
14. Drob, S, Loemer, M and Lifshutz, H. Genital herpes: the psychological consequences. *British Journal of Medical Psychology*, 1985: 307–315.
15. Macgregor, J. *Herpes: the latest word*. Melbourne: Currey O'Neil, 1983.

CHAPTER 12

LEGAL AND ETHICAL CONSIDERATIONS

Schover and Jensen[1] outline professional issues which are likely to arise when the medical practitioner takes sexual histories and provides sexual counselling.

Confidentiality

While confidentiality is necessary in all medical practice, it is of paramount importance when matters of an intensely personal and private nature are discussed. You need to make every effort to ensure that information about sexuality is shared by the physician and patient alone.

Schover and Jensen suggest that practitioners working in an institutional setting seek special permission to keep private notes only on sexual matters. Ward and outpatient notes are of necessity easily accessible to a wide range of health professionals and health professional students. We would suggest that it is perhaps even more important in the general practice setting, where notes may be accessible to non-professional persons. Especially in a country setting, it is quite possible that secretaries and receptionists will know patients socially.

We have seen a further issue of confidentiality in couples therapy when one partner has initially seen the practitioner alone (see chapter five). It is essential that the consultation start from square one, with both partners having their say. The initial patient may well have told the practitioner information which he or she has not discussed with the partner. Not only would it perhaps cause dissension, but it would underscore the worry of the second partner that the therapist and patient one are in an unholy alliance. If you are in any doubt at all, discuss what may be revealed to the partner before the couples session takes place.

If at all possible, the patient's permission should be sought before the case is discussed with colleagues.

The seductive patient

In any doctor–patient setting, the potential exists for the patient to behave seductively. Research suggests that a proportion of medical practitioners make positive responses to sexual advances. Some even claim that in psychiatric practice it may be therapeutic.[2] We take the stand that sexual intercourse with patients represents an exploitation of the doctor–patient relationship and should simply never be allowed to occur. Registration boards similarly tend to frown on sexual relations with patients and ex-patients.

What then should you do? Simply ignoring sexual innuendo or physical advances is unlikely to solve the problem. Box 12A gives an example of acknowledgement of the patient's advance, gentle rejection of it and a firm re-establishment of the doctor–patient relationship on a professional footing.

Schover and Jensen give guidelines for handling seductive or acting-out patients. They are outlined in Box 12B.

BOX 12A

The seductive patient

First year medical students watched a video vignette and were asked how they would respond. They saw an earthily attractive woman aged about 18, who had returned for a check up on an infected foot. She looked, rather fiercely, directly at the camera and said, 'I don't know how to say this, but I really like you. I think you're great.'

An extremely good-looking male student, presumably well used to dealing with such advances gave this response. 'It's really nice of you to say that. Thanks. Now let's have a look at that foot.'

This reply graciously acknowledges the advance, defuses it and then returns the consultation to a professional basis.

Consent

The patient has every right to refuse to talk about sexuality.
There are three defining characteristics of informed consent:

- The patient should be told sufficient details about what is being agreed to and any risks involved.

- The patient should be capable of understanding what he or she is told. (Capability is often defined in terms of age, intellectual capacity or psychiatric state.)
- The patient should not be coerced in any way into giving consent.

Perhaps the last characteristic is most important here. Even though the practitioner firmly believes that it it is the best interests of the patient to discuss sexuality, he or she must be ready to drop the topic at once if the patient shows reluctance. It is enough simply to have made it clear that sexuality is an O.K. topic and thereby leave the door open for discussion in the future if the patient sees fit.

BOX 12B

Guidelines for treating seductive patients

- Try to understand the patient's motivation in making the advance.
- Try not to react angrily. This will severely damage the doctor–patient relationship.
- Explore the meaning of the advance to the patient in a counselling framework.
- Consult with senior colleagues if you feel out of your depth.
- When working with patients with a history of sexual aggression, make sure the consultation takes place where the assistance of other people is easily available.

Schover and Jensen, 1988

How much do you need to know?

Patients may perceive questions about sexuality as voyeuristic, especially when they have presented for diagnosis or treatment of a physical illness. The 'normalising' approach that states that many patients with that particular illness find that they are having sexual problems (see chapter five) may overcome the difficulty.

Nonetheless, it is essential that questions about sexuality be asked only where they are related to the patient's welfare rather than the prurient curiosity of the practitioner.

> **BOX 12C**
>
> ## A doctor's dilemma
>
> Stephen is a 46-year old homosexual man. He has never had a steady sexual relationship and his sexual activities have been with casual partners and pick-ups only.
>
> In July 1985 he was diagnosed as HIV-positive and counselled about safe sex practices. He attended only one of the three counselling appointments given to him.
>
> In subsequent consultations he said that he usually practised safe sex except on a few occasions. This was 'not much'. He rejected zidovudine therapy in favour of herbal remedies.
>
> Since 1973 he had been presenting to the STD clinic with a variety of STD-related and non-STD problems. Since 1982, when he presented with a severe episode of herpes zoster, some if not all of the presentations could be related to HIV infection.
>
> He remained remarkably physically well and up to October 1990 suffered no notable weight loss despite significant reductions in T4 cells and T4:T8 ratio.
>
> In July 1990 Karposi's sarcoma was diagnosed on biopsy. When the biopsy specimen was being taken he asked, 'You don't think it's cancer, do you, doc?' He was told that the biopsy was meant to find that out and he declined to ask further questions.
>
> A colleague who visited Stephen some four weeks after the diagnosis of Kaposi's sarcoma found that he was planning a massive reorganisation of his garden and a protracted overseas trip.
>
> His doctor at the clinic felt that he was using denial as a coping mechanism for the following reasons:
>
> - His reluctance to ask questions or discuss his condition.
> - His lack of curiosity about his condition.
> - His continued occasional unsafe sex.
> - The unrealistic nature of his plans for the future.
> - His rejection of zidovudine therapy.
>
> The question was whether to make attempts to break through that denial. This might have had the public health advantage of discouraging him from unsafe sexual practices. His denial was also possibly a factor in his rejection of the preferred medical treatment. On the other hand, it is impossible to predict the mental and physical consequences of breaking down denial, especially given rather limited information about his premorbid coping style.
>
> Bassett, 1990

Ethical issues in sexually-transmitted diseases

Almond[3] was talking with specific reference to AIDS when she characterised two different and often conflicting ideologies with regard to ethical issues in sexually-transmitted diseases.

- **Civil liberties:** The right of the individual not to be subjected to potential discrimination because of public knowledge that he or she has a sexually-transmitted disease.
- **Public health:** The right of the community to protection from the spread of sexually-transmitted diseases.

Box 12C gives a case history where a doctor found herself in something of a dilemma resulting from the conflicting modes of action derived from these two positions.

Crisp[4] focuses specifically on situations where the doctor faces a moral dilemma between respecting the interests of the patient and those of the community. His examples include:

- The patient who refuses to give up high risk behaviours.
- The patient who has asked not to be told the results of HIV testing and who tests positive.
- The HIV-positive person who refuses to tell the sexual partner.
- The doctor who wishes not to treat an HIV-positive patient.
- The possible use of a blood sample taken to confirm a diagnosis of anaemia in an anonymous research programme to collect statistics on HIV prevalence.
- The HIV-positive doctor who intends not to reveal the fact to patients.

Crisp gives alternative courses of action that the practitioner might take, but concludes that it is the personal balance of importance of the two conflicting ideals which will determine the course taken.

Legal issues

The legal aspects of taking a sexual history and sexual counselling must also be considered. While these may change across jurisdictions, there are a number of common elements which the practitioner must be aware of. These relate to the legal obligations of the practitioner to notify particular categories of diseases, to carry out counselling with regard to particular diseases, and to disclose particular matters to the authorities. Further, the practitioner should be aware of the legal complexities of assault, confidentiality and consent.

Notification of disease

In almost all jurisdictions, particular diseases are notifiable to the authorities (usually the Department of Health) to aid in establishing the range and magnitude of disease in the community. Invariably these include sexually transmissible diseases (particularly HIV, gonorrhoea, syphilis, and chlamydia, although this will differ from jurisdiction to jurisdiction). If a proven case of disease is diagnosed, then this is usually notifiable by name and with other identifying details. In the case of presumptive disease which is treated without definitive proof (for example, without laboratory confirmation) the situation is less clear-cut, and the practitioner should seek the advice of the local health department on the criteria necessary for notification. There are usually special forms for notification, and the information is held confidentially and does not go beyond the officer to whom it is notified.

Disclosure

Disclosure of information to a third party should always be confirmed by obtaining written consent from the patient (with the exception of those disclosures required by law). However, there may be a number of difficult situations in which this is not possible. For example, if the practitioner treats both spouses or partners and is aware that one has had sex outside the relationship, yet is forbidden to convey this information to the other partner, then this instruction must be followed.

This situation is complicated when the infection which has occurred is a potentially fatal one (eg, HIV infection). The legal situation has been complicated by several cases in the United States in which it has been held that if a person is in danger (the classic case was of danger from a psychotic patient who had indicated their intent to kill someone), then the practitioner has a duty to warn the person in danger. Just how far this can be generalised is uncertain, as is its application outside the United States. Generally, the safest option is to assume that in the absence of permission, the threat must be a major and immediate one before confidentiality can be broken. Disclosure raises a conflict between the duty of confidentiality and the duty to protect third parties against foreseeable transmission of disease or other harm. It must be realised that possible consequences of disclosure may include discrimination, stigmatisation and ostracism. In the area of HIV infection, Landsell[6] comprehensively reviews the issues which arise and in particular the legal duties in various jurisdictions. She notes that conflicts may easily arise between the individual's right to privacy and the interest of public health, safety and welfare. In general, unless the danger is foreseeable and direct (that is, there is a specific danger to a particular individual rather than a broadly anticipated one), disclosure is not justified. That is, confidentiality is the rule unless there are extremely compelling reasons otherwise. However, there are exceptions to this in the realm of the criminal law.

Criminal law: Where the patient has committed a crime, then the practitioner should report this to the appropriate authorities. There is no recognition of confidentiality by the law where crime (as opposed to the civil law) is involved. Thus, if there is evidence of sexual assault, sex with a minor, or any other criminal situation, the practitioner has an obligation to report this to the appropriate authorities. Similarly, when the courts require (in respect of a criminal matter) that the practitioner provide notes or other documents, then the practitioner is obliged to supply these (regardless of whether the patient has given permission or not). Note here the distinction made between the **criminal** law (which concerns matters which are crimes as defined in the criminal law) and the **civil** law (which concerns matters such as damages, contracts, and so on).

Improper conduct with patients

This area has both ethical (as already noted) and legal aspects. What is considered **unethical** may not necessarily be **illegal** (for example, sexual contact with a consenting patient). However, examination of a patient (particularly a genital examination) may be considered an assault if there is not a clear assent for the examination to occur. It is useful to spell out beforehand what is to be done and what it will involve. Clearly, the boundary between examination and assault is nebulous and from time to time patients do take their practitioners to court charging assault: this is usually in regard to genital or breast examination. It is wise to make sure that there is at least some other staff member in the building (although not necessarily in the room) when carrying out a genital examination and if in doubt, it is useful to have another health practitioner present or close by.

The issue of obtaining consent for specific tests (the most obvious case being HIV tests) is more clouded. This depends on whether the practitioner has got a blanket approval for 'some tests' or whether the tests have been specified. In general, it is wise to specify the tests involved and opinion is divided over whether taking a test such as an HIV test without permission may constitute an assault. In some jurisdictions, the law provides that HIV tests may not be done without counselling and thus carrying out a test without such counselling carries legal penalties.

We have already noted that sexual contact with a patient is considered unethical. If this does occur, it may provide grounds for a civil action against the practitioner by the spouse, or action to de-register the practitioner for improper conduct. Generally, registration boards, medical colleges and other professional societies take a dim view of such conduct and de-registration or withdrawal of a licence to practice, or some other censure, may result. Thus, unethical conduct, while not specifically illegal, may have legal consequences.

Seeking advice

Where one is in doubt, one should seek advice. Many situations regarding ethics and the law are complex and involve weighing up a number of arguments for and against particular actions. Unless immediate action is necessary, it is strongly advisable to at least confer with a senior colleague, and if possible to seek the advice of one's professional or registering body. In many cases, one has to weigh up the legal and ethical issues, which will not necessarily be congruent. For example, the issue of maintaining confidentiality seems to outweigh the legal requirement to notify a crime, or vice versa. In such cases, consultation with senior colleagues is mandatory and will frequently clarify the issue without involving the practitioner in contentious situations. When in any doubt, consult.

References

1. Schover, L.R and Jensen, S.B. *Sexuality and chronic illness. A comprehensive approach.* New York: The Guilford Press, 1988.
2. Carr, M and Robinson, G.E. Fatal attraction: the ethical and clinical dilemma of patient–therapist sex. *Canadian Journal of Psychiatry*, 1990: 35, 122–127.

3. Almond, B. (ed.) *AIDS–a moral issue. The ethical, legal and social aspects.* London: Macmillan, 1990.
4. Crisp, R. *Autonomy, welfare and the treatment of AIDS.* In B. Almond (ed.) *AIDS–a moral issue. The ethical, legal and social aspects.* London: Macmillan, 1990.
5. Bassett, I. Personal communication, 1990.
6. Landsell, G.T. AIDS, the law and civil liberties. *Medical Journal of Australia*, 1991, 154: 61–67.

CHAPTER 13

UNDERSTANDING AND COUNSELLING: THE HOMOSEXUAL PATIENT

The issue of seeing patients with different sexual lifestyles from the majority of people one sees concerns many practitioners, if only at the level of knowledge. It is important to emphasise the fact that there is probably no typical 'homosexual' patient any more than there is a typical 'heterosexual' patient. On the other hand, there are a number of aspects of homosexual lifestyles which differ from many aspects of heterosexual lifestyles. These are discussed in an attempt to clarify the appropriate medical and professional approach to homosexual individuals who may be patients.

It is equally important to note that until the last few years, sexual medicine courses were not available in medical schools with the result that medical practitioners have little, if any, knowledge about homosexuality over and above that held by the educated layperson. For this reason, it is important firstly to define homosexuality and to place it into a medical context.

The homosexual–heterosexual continuum

Contrary to popular opinion, 'homosexuals' and 'heterosexuals' do not comprise two separate classes of people. Kinsey and colleagues[1] noted that individuals fit into a continuum which has exclusive heterosexuality at one end and exclusive homosexuality at the other.[1] If one considers that one in three male patients is likely to have had a homosexual experience leading to orgasm between the ages of 16 and 65 years, and that almost one in five will have had as much homosexual experience as heterosexual for at least a three-year period in the same age range, then it is clear that the world cannot be divided into homosexuals and heterosexuals. However, because our society does stigmatise homosexual relations, we tend to divide individuals arbitrarily into 'homosexuals' and 'heterosexuals' and assume that these are absolute classes. In this book we define 'homosexual' as predominantly homosexual at a particular point in time.

Homosexual preference may be primary, i.e. having sex is more important than who it is with, or secondary, i.e. the emotional attraction is to the same sex as well. Thus individuals may be behaviourally homosexual but not emotionally or vice versa. It is important to differentiate practice from preference. As an example, McConaghy and colleagues[2] found that over 40% were aware of homosexual feelings, although presumably a much smaller percentage would have acted on these feelings. Within so-called 'homosexual' male samples, Saghir and Robins[3] found that over 48% had had sexual relations with a woman which, as well as illustrating the lack of discrete groups, points to the fact that male homosexuality is not a distaste for female sexual partners but a preference for male ones.

Disclosure and medical attitudes

Those patients who indicate to their medical practitioner that they are homosexual will do so for a variety of reasons, either because they wish to discuss the area with regard to sexual counselling[4] or because they believe that this information will aid medical management. However, not all overtly homosexual patients will share the fact of their sexual preference. Dardick and Grady[5] found that less than 50% of openly homosexual men in the US had told their primary health-care provider that they were gay. One must assume that for those who are covertly homosexual the figure is even lower. In Australia, over 20% of gay men presenting with sexually transmitted diseases did not tell the attending practitioner that their infection was homosexually acquired.[6] Unfortunately, one of the reasons for this is that three-quarters of a sample of 1000 doctors acknowledged that knowing a male patient was homosexual would adversely affect their medical management.[7] As recently as 1980, 84% of American physicians surveyed agreed that homosexual patients hesitate to seek health care because of physician disapproval.[8]

More recently, Davison and Friedman[9] found that when two groups of psychologists were given a case history of a male, and one group was told incidentally that the patient was homosexual, most of the patient's problems were construed by that group in sexual terms, and the sexual aspect concentrated on. It would appear that emotional biases, usually activated by lack of reliable information, may adversely affect medical treatment and patient counselling. Compounding this is the problem that while the general practitioner is usually the individual to whom problems of a sexual nature are first taken, sexual medicine is only now being included in medical school curricula. Unless practitioners have sufficient information on homosexuality to avoid falling back into personal reactions or invoking popular stereotypes, they are best advised to avoid counselling homosexual patients.

In light of this, it is important to realise that if a male patient volunteers information about his homosexuality the decision has probably not been taken lightly, and that an understanding and accepting response is important. It is also important not to assume that all patients are heterosexual unless one is advised to the contrary. Indeed, between 10% and 20% of gay men are or have been heterosexually married,[4] and some 54% of homosexual encounters in public conveniences are by married men who define themselves as heterosexual.[10]

Areas of difference in homosexual health care

When a male patient has revealed his sexual orientation, this is usually in the interests of honesty and obtaining more complete health care. There is a tendency to see a homosexual preference as pertaining only to sexual matters, which is a particularly narrow definition. While this information may mean swabbing of additional sites for sexually transmissible diseases if the patient is sexually active (anorectal as well as the usual urethral and oropharyngeal sites), it also has farther reaching implications.

Since a homosexual preference is still stigmatised to a greater or lesser extent in Australasian society, the patient will carry burdens associated with either coping with negative reaction if he is overtly homosexual or, if he is not openly homosexual, coping with the anxieties of keeping sexual orientation hidden and fear of disclosure. The cost of this will be extremely variable. However, there are considerable implications in terms of psychosomatic illness including unexplained headaches, hypertension, gastrointestinal disorders ranging from ulceration to irritable bowel syndrome, and asthma which has a functional component. Psychological stress may also present in a variety of less somatic forms, such as sleep disturbance or generalised anxiety. In most cases the stress is manageable through an accepting clinical interaction or referral to stress management programmes and relaxation training.

On the other hand, the great majority of homosexual men will experience little or no problems with their sexual orientation. It is important to note that homosexuality has not been considered a mental disorder since it was removed from the Descriptive and Statistical Manual (DSM–III) of the American Psychiatric Association in 1973. Nor is there any evidence that, as a group, homosexuals are any different to heterosexuals in their psychological stability and mental functioning. Apart from difficulties with the same range of problems which trouble heterosexual individuals, the homosexual patient may be remarkable in psychological terms only where stigma management presents as an issue.

Ego-dystonic homosexuality, where an individual is homosexual but does not want to be, or is disturbed by being homosexual, is however listed. While there is a great deal of evidence that sexual preference does not imply psychological maladjustment, where a sexual preference is devalued by the society either legally, religiously or socially, there will be more problems associated with it. Most counselling of homosexuals, apart from general problems which face all individuals, relates to management of stigma.

In some cases, the patient may have internalised this stigma to the extent where they see as a solution the removal of their homosexual orientation.

Behaviour modification, however, is not successful in this regard, since predominantly homosexual individuals are able to make only a very limited heterosexual adjustment, which is usually not sustainable over time. It is far better to counsel toward self-acceptance.[11] Some writers have argued that one cures only diseases, and that since attempting to remove homosexual behaviour is simply enforcing a societal moral judgement on patients who do not come of their own free will (given the stigma attached to their sexual orientation), it is unethical to attempt to do so.[12] From the point of view of the general practitioner, it is important to be aware that patient requests to modify sexual preference may reflect problems of stigma management and be symptomatic of difficulties more amenable to counselling, rather than to take the patient's request at face value. It is also necessary to differentiate a homosexual preference from core or marginal transvestism or transsexualism. A few homosexuals may request gender reassignment in order to make their same-sex desires 'legitimate' by becoming a member of the 'opposite sex'.

Stages of acceptance of homosexuality

Patients will present in different stages of their homosexuality. The best model for describing the path to acceptance of one's sexual orientation has been described by Cass.[13] She has posited six stages in the development of a homosexual identity in the individual:

1. Identity confusion
2. Identity comparison
3. Identity tolerance
4. Identity acceptance
5. Identity pride
6. Identity synthesis.

Identity confusion describes the stage where individuals feel that they are different from others and that their feelings or behaviours may be labelled as homosexual. The second stage, identity comparison, is where the individual makes the first tentative commitment to a homosexual identity and the realisation of being homosexual to a degree.

With identity tolerance in the individual comes the recognition that he or she is probably homosexual and a degree of commitment to this identity arises. By stage four, the identity acceptance stage, the individual accepts the label of homosexual, at least in gay company, and begins to socialise within a gay subculture. The stage of identity pride is marked by wide disclosure and open activism and describes the situation where everything the individual does is defined primarily by his or her homosexuality. At this stage, the central identity of the person is as a homosexual.

The sixth stage of the Cass model is perhaps the one which has stimulated most debate. In the individual, the 'them versus us' view of homosexuals and heterosexuals fades, and is replaced by a situation where the person's homosexual identity is seen as being one of a series of identities, but not one which defines all aspects of the person's lifestyle. The individual may thus see being homosexual as an incidental matter like political belief or occupation, and not something that he or she is all the time.

It is important that we deal with patients' sexuality depending on the level of acceptance they are at and do not try to push them too fast through these stages. We should let them achieve these stages, with encouragement, at their own pace.

Homosexual relationships

The popular view of the homosexual as promiscuous is not an accurate one for the great majority of gay individuals. A recent survey of gay men in the US found that the median number of lifetime sexual partners of sexually continuously active individuals was less than 50.[14] It is important to bear this in mind when reading of atypical samples (e.g. many AIDS cases) in which numbers of sexual partners may number in the hundreds or thousands.

A significant proportion of gay men and women will be in homosexual relationships. These relationships have been classified into four general categories in a study by Bell and Weinberg.[15] They divided their sample into:

1. Close-coupleds
2. Open-coupleds
3. Functionals
4. Dysfunctionals.

The 'close-coupleds' were closely bound together and monogamous, in the sense that the two individuals tended to look to one another for sexual and interpersonal satisfactions. They had the lowest level of sexual or psychological problems.

The 'open-coupleds' were living with a special sexual partner, but tended to seek sexual interpersonal satisfactions with people outside their partnership although this tended to worry them. Psychologically and sexually, they had no more or less problems than other groups.

The 'functionals' were the equivalent of the swinging singles, and appeared to organise their life around their sexual experiences. They tended to have wide social circles and few sexual and psychological problems.

In contrast, the 'dysfunctionals' were troubled people whose life offered them little gratification and who displayed significantly greater psychological and sexual problems than any other group. This group most closely accorded with the old stereotype of the tormented homosexual.

While this sketch of homosexual relational patterns is brief, it does indicate the great diversity of interpersonal styles which exist within a homosexual life-style.

Sexual practices and sexually transmissible diseases

To most people, it is sexual practices and gender of partner which sets homosexuals apart from heterosexuals. In practice, however, the same range of sexual activities are practised by both heterosexuals and homosexuals, with the exception of penovaginal intercourse in homosexuals. It is not generally realised that anal receptive intercourse is practised regularly by one in twelve women.[16] While some homosexual men do have a preference for a particular role in anal intercourse or fellatio, the most common situation is for multiple sexual activities to occur in any sexual interaction.

Contrary to popular opinion, anal intercourse only occurs in about one third of male homosexual encounters. Fellatio and mutual masturbation are more common in terms of frequency.[17] In homosexual women, activities will most commonly involve oral or manual stimulation.

From a medical point of view, anal intercourse if carried out with inadequate lubrication or any great degree of vigour may lead to lesions of the rectal epithelium which in places may be thin in contrast to the cornified vaginal epithelium. This may act as a portal for pathogens, and thus lead to greater risk than with penovaginal intercourse. The range of sexually transmissible diseases associated with homosexual men includes syphilis, gonorrhoea, non-gonococcal urethritis, hepatitis (A, B, and C), herpes, and the so-called 'gay bowel syndrome' including infections, anal warts and proctitis.[18]

Sexual attitudes affect lifestyle

While hepatitis and enteric infections are associated with analingus, a practice apparently much more common in the US than in Australasia, it is important to note that the spectrum of sexually transmissible diseases is markedly broader in sexually active homosexual men than was traditionally assumed. To these sexually transmissible diseases must now be added AIDS.

While the greater majority of homosexual men will not be at any greater risk of sexually related infections than heterosexual men, it is important to expand our previously narrow view of the range of sexually transmissible diseases and to test for additional pathogens in homosexually active men where symptoms occur. As an example, some 37% of Australasian homosexually active men may be surface antibody positive for hepatitis B.[19]

Attitudes to sexuality and risk factors in homosexual men

In a recent study of the psychological and social factors which influence sexually transmitted disease risks, it was found that particular dimensions of sexual attitudes best predicted how the individual managed a homosexual lifestyle.[17] These dimensions included attitudes to relationships, degree of control of sexual excitement and libido, degree of being visually stimulated by members of the same gender, social comfort, acceptance of one's homosexuality, and degree of permissiveness or prudishness. Homosexual individuals may vary across all of these dimensions. It would be a mistake to assume that the simple fact of a homosexual preference can predict anything about how the individual exists as a homosexual. Again it must also be emphasised that the range of attitudes in homosexual men and women is as wide as the range of attitudes in heterosexual men and women. However, those attitudinal dimensions referred to above do appear to be the important ones in determining what sort of sexual lifestyle is led.

Homosexual women

Homosexual women are at much less risk than heterosexual women of contracting sexually transmissible diseases[20] and also enjoy on average much better mental health than heterosexual women.[21] They may still present with the usual range of medical problems as other women, although these are unlikely to be directly related to their sexual preference. Most if not all of the comments made with regard to male homosexuals will also apply to dealing with female homosexual patients, although some of the difficulties faced by homosexual women may include issues such as childrearing. There may also be difficulties with the management of social stigma.

Counselling approaches

When an individual reveals his or her homosexuality to the medical practitioner, it is usually for one or two reasons. Firstly, to give the practitioner information which may be necessary in health care (for diverse reasons such as transmission of sexually related diseases to informing the practitioner that somebody the patient has lived with for 20 years is next of kin), and secondly, to raise issues or problems associated with homosexuality. In many cases, the first comment about sexual preference will be to test the practitioner's response, and uncertainty or negativity usually preclude the matter being raised again. Gentle inquiry as to whether being homosexual has caused any problems may elicit further details if they are not forthcoming. It should be borne in mind that the decision to reveal a homosexual orientation has usually been turned over in the mind numerous times, and that several visits may need to be made before an opportunity presents itself for the patient to discuss the matter. On the other hand, some patients will deny their sexual orientation if asked.

In many cases, the homosexual orientation becomes the subject of concern, rather than the complaint about homosexuality being seen as symptomatic of other problems. For example, Serber and Keith[22] found that the reason their patients were dissatisfied with being homosexual and wanted to become heterosexual was because they were lonely and isolated as homosexuals. Following a course of training in social skills and assertiveness, the patients were able to interact socially with other homosexuals, and they reported that they were happy with their sexual preference and would not want to become heterosexuals even if this were possible. Bell[23] comments in this regard that 'I am homosexual' is not self-explanatory, and such a declaration means different things to and about different people. Only after exhaustive discussion by the patient of his or her position with respect to the various dimensions of homosexual experience can a more complete picture emerge.

Thus it is necessary to determine whether the problem is related to being unable to function adequately as a homosexual, or to problems brought on by being homosexual. This latter group includes individuals being unsure if they are homosexual, negative reactions from family, employers or peers, marital or relationship difficulties, and in some states where homosexual behaviour is still proscribed, legal charges.

'Coming out'

'Coming out', as an individual's acceptance of his or her homosexuality is known, is probably one of the most stressful moments in which counselling may be sought, particularly as at this stage the support of other homosexuals is not available and the individual may not only feel that he or she is the 'only one in the world' but also have no information about homosexuality apart from the public myths and stereotypes. What is most necessary, given that the person has usually become fairly certain over a period of several years that he or she is homosexual before confiding in others, is to be able to direct the patient's attention to those areas which will clarify the degree of homosexuality, and to sources of information on homosexuals. Frequently individuals cannot identify themselves as homosexual because they did not fit the public stereotype (e.g. being effeminate), or because they also have some degree of heterosexual interest. Conversely, individuals who have little or no same-sex interest may become anxious if they do not fit the conventional masculine or feminine stereotype, and counselling should follow a similar course.

First it is essential to avoid value judgements about sexual preference and avoid giving the impression of disapproval if the individual is to be helped to make an honest judgement. Secondly, information regarding homosexuality and the spectrum of sexual variation must be presented for the individual to be able to make his or her own differential diagnosis as to sexual preference. Thirdly, if it is necessary for patients to make contact with other homosexuals, in order to establish their affinity or otherwise, then this should also be encouraged. This is the PLISSIT model,[24] which is a general model of sexual counselling — the letters stand for Permission, Limited Information, Specific Suggestion, and Intensive Therapy. The general practitioner can progress to the third stage leaving the final stage to an appropriately qualified specialist. Initially, permission for the patient to be homosexual must be given, or acceptance indicated — in some cases this will be sufficient to enable resolution of the problem. This may be followed by limited information which may help place the problem in context or suggest ways of resolving it. Following this, it may occasionally be necessary for the practitioner to make specific suggestions as to actions the patient may take or experiment with. It has been found that up to 80% of general sexual problems can resolve this way, and it offers a useful guide to counselling the homosexual.

Common problems

Common difficulties with which homosexuals present include reactions of family and peers which are negative (these sometimes may be resolved by counselling the family using the first two stages of the model), and the more complex problem of homosexuality within marriage. While this is a complicated subject[4] and cannot be treated in a generalised fashion, counselling should aim to define the degree of homosexuality and the point to which compromise is possible.

Similarly, it is often as difficult to advise on methods of counselling relationship difficulties in homosexual couples as it is to advise on the vast range of marital difficulties. What is essential is to determine whether the patient's homosexuality is bound up in the problem which requires counselling or whether the homosexual preference is essentially unrelated to it, and not let the patient's sexuality become a central issue when it is not a cause of the problem.

In conclusion, the requirements for successful counselling of homosexual patients, given that the range of problems requiring counselling in heterosexuals as well as homosexuals is probably infinite, include a lack of prejudgement and sufficient knowledge of the area to provide information and perspectives the homosexual patient may be lacking, and suggestions for specific action. Added to this base, a mutually agreed upon goal, if counselling is likely to be extended, and a model within which to structure the therapy are important. While the counselling skills needed on the part of the practitioner are the same as those needed for other patients, genuineness, non-possessive warmth and accurate empathy,[25] it is important that the view of individuals as being *either* homosexual *or* heterosexual is not reinforced, and that the individuality of the patient is not submerged under this one aspect of their lifestyle. The ultimate goal of counselling should be for patients to accept their sexual preference, but not define their whole existence in terms of it.

Conclusion

In conclusion, while it is important to have a medical and psychological understanding of the range of problems which homosexual men and women may have, it is also critical that we see these health problems as being neither solely sexually related nor stereotypically homosexual. In understanding and managing homosexual patients, the central issue is to appreciate that homosexual individuals cover the same wide spectrum of humanity as heterosexual persons, and that the division of people into 'heterosexual' and 'homosexual' groups is arbitrary although less psychologically threatening. The ultimate management mistake is to see patients in terms of their homosexuality alone and to ignore the fact that their sexual orientation may be a minor aspect of their identity and personality. The diversity of individuals who may be homosexual precludes generalisation about them from the fact of their sexual orientation alone.

References

1. Kinsey, A.C, Pomeroy, W.B and Martin, C.E. *Sexual behavior in the human male*. Philadelphia: W.B. Saunders, 1948.
2. McConaghy, N, Armstrong, N, Birrell, P.C and Buhrich, N. The incidence of bisexual feelings and opposite sex behavior in medical students. *Journal of Nervous and Mental Disease*, 1979: 167, 685–688.
3. Saghir, M.T and Robins, E. *Male and female homosexuality: a comprehensive investigation*. Baltimore: Williams & Wilkins, 1973.
4. Ross, M.W. *The married homosexual man: a psychological study*. London: Routledge and Kegan Paul, 1983.
5. Dardick, L and Grady, D. Openness between gay persons and health professionals. *Ann Intern Med*, 1980: 93, 115–119.
6. Ross, M.W. Attitudes of male homosexuals to venereal disease clinics. *Med J Aust*, 1981: 2, 670–671.
7. Pauly, I.B and Goldstein, S. Physician's attitudes in treating homosexuals. *Medical Aspects of Human Sexuality*, 1970: 4, 26–45.
8. Sandholzer, T.A. Physician attitudes and other factors affecting the incidence of sexually transmitted diseases in homosexual men. *Journal of Homosexuality*, 1980: 5, 325–327.
9. Davison, G.C and Friedman, S. Sexual orientation stereotype in the distortion of clinical judgement. *Journal of Homosexuality*, 1981: 6(3), 37–44.
10. Humphreys, R.A.Z. *Tearoom trade: a study of impersonal sex in public places*. London: Duckworth, 1970.
11. Freund, K. Should homosexuality arouse therapeutic concern? *Journal of Homosexuality*, 1977: 2, 235–240.
12. Davison, G.C. Homosexuality: the ethical challenge. *Journal of Consulting and Clinical Psychology*, 1976: 44, 157–162.
13. Cass, V.C. Homosexual identity formation: a theoretical model. *Journal of Homosexuality*, 1979: 4, 219–235.
14. Darrow, W.W, Barrett, D, Jay, K and Young, A. The gay report on sexually transmitted diseases. *Am J Public Health*, 1981: 71, 1004–1011.
15. Bell, A.P and Weinberg, M.S. *Homosexualities: a study of diversity among men and women*. Melbourne: Macmillan, 1978.
16. Bolling, D.R. Prevalence, goals and complications of heterosexual anal intercourse in a gynaecologic population. *Journal of Reproductive Medicine*, 1977: 19, 120–124.
17. Ross, M.W. *Psychovenereology: personality and lifestyle factors in sexually transmitted diseases in homosexual men*. New York: Praeger, 1986.
18. Ostrow, D.G and Altman, N.L. Sexually transmitted diseases and homosexuality. *Sex Transm Dis*, 1981: 8, 75–76.
19. Burrell, C.J, Cameron, A.S, Hart, G. Melbourne, J and Beal, R.W. Hepatitis B reservoirs and attack rates in an Australian community. *Med J Aust*, 1983: 2, 492–496.
20. Robertson, P and Schacter, J. Failure to identify venereal disease in a lesbian population. *Sex Transm Dis*, 1981: 8, 75–76.
21. Freedman, M. *Homosexuality and psychological functioning*. Belmont: Brooks-Cole, 1971.
22. Serber, M and Keith, C.G. The Atascadero project: model of a sexual retraining program for incarcerated homosexual pedophiles. *Journal of Homosexuality*, 1974: 1, 87–97.

23. Bell, A.P. The homosexual as patient. In: Green, R. (ed.) *Human sexuality: a health practitioner's text*. (2nd edn). Baltimore: Williams & Wilkins, 1979: 98–114.
24. Annon, J.S. *The behavioral treatment of sexual problems: brief therapy*. Honolulu: Enabling Systems, 1974.
25. Truax, C.B & Carkhuff, R.R. *Toward effective counselling and psychotherapy: training and practice*. Chicago: Aldine, 1967.

INDEX

A

AIDS
    staging reactions to 80–4
    see also HIV
anal intercourse 37
anorgasmia 22–4
    treatments 57–61
anticholinergic agents 101
antihypertensives 101

B

behavioural counselling 42–3

C

cancer 90–1
    self examination for 91–2
central nervous system depressants 100–1
chronic illness 94, 85
    psychosocial effects of 96
'coming out' 139–40
condom
    and contraception 39
contact tracing 39–40
contraception 88–9
counselling, general 42–7
    PLISSIT model 48–9
    see also STD counselling; sexual dysfunction
couples therapy 43–4
    see also sexual dysfunction

D

drugs 92–3
    anticholinergic agents 101
    antihypertensives 101
    central nervous system depressants 100–1
    hormones 102
    opioids 101
    prolactin stimulators 101–2
    social drugs 102–3
dyspareunia 32

E

ego-dystonic homosexuality 134
emotional difficulties
    and sexual histories 11–12
empathy 14–16
erectile dysfunction 29, 30
    treatments 51–3
ethical issues 129
    civil liberties 125, 126
    confidentiality 122
    consent 123–4
    improper conduct 128–9

G

Goldman's rule 13

H

herpes
    lifestyle implications 79

herpes
    psychological associations 78–9, 79–80
HIV
    consent 109–10
    coping mechanisms 107–8
    preventive behaviour 110
    reaction to the test 107
    reasons for testing 106
    recording test results 111–12
    risk behaviours 106–7
    staging reactions to 80–4
    support structures 108–9
    testing for 104–5, 110–11
    homosexual–heterosexual continuum 131–2
homosexual patient, understanding 141–2
    common problems 140–1
    counselling approaches 138–9
    ego-dystonic homosexuality 134
    health care requirements 133–4
    practitioner attitudes to 132–3
    stages in acceptance 135
    and STD risks 137–8
homosexual relationships 136
    risk factors in men 138
    risk factors in women 138
    and STDs 137–8
hormones 102

I

infertility 62–4
    counselling support 64–6
informed consent 109–10
intercourse history
    men's 27–32
    women's 19

K

Kinsey's rule 13

L

language, in history taking 12–14
legal issues 129
    confidentiality 35, 122
    consent 123–4
    criminal law issues 128
    disease notification 127
    disclosure 127–8
    improper conduct 128–9

M

manual sex 38
marital difficulties
    and sexual histories 11–12
Masters and Johnson squeeze technique 55
men
    taking sexual history 27–32
menstruation, questions about 18
Mitford's rule 14

N

notification, of STDs 35
    disease notification 127
    partners 39–40

O

obstetric history 18–19
opioids 101
oral sex 38
Orwell's rule 13–14

P

PLISSIT model 48–9
post-test HIV counselling 112
    for negative results 112–13
    for positive results 113–20

practitioner embarrassment 3, 4
pre-test HIV counselling 104–10
premature ejaculation 29–30, 31
    treatments, 53–6
preventative education 2
preventive health care 88
    cancer 90–1
    contraception 88–9
    STD 89
    prolactin stimulators 101–2
psychiatric illness
    effects on sexuality 94–6

R

referral 49
    in HIV 119
relationships, current
    in men 27–8
    in women 20
retarded ejaculation 30–2
    treatments 56–7
Rogers, Carl 42

S

screening histories 8–9
    in men 9
    reasons for 20
    in women 9
seductive patients, dealing with 123, 124
self-examination for cancer 91–2
Semans' technique 55
sensate focus exercises 50–7
sex toys 92
sexual behaviours
    in women 20–1
sexual discounting 2
sexual dysfunction, men 28
    and chronic illness 94–8
    and drugs 101–3
    dyspareunia 32
    erectile dysfunction 29, 30
    premature ejaculation 29–30, 31
    retarded ejaculation 30–2
    treatments 50–7
sexual dysfunction, women 23, 24–5
    anorgasmia 22–4
    and chronic illness 94–8
    and drugs 101–3
    treatments 57–62
    vaginismus 25–6
sexual history-taking 12
    emotional difficulties and 11–12
    empathy with patient 14
    failure to take 3–4, 8
    gender assumptions 38–9
    from lesbian women 22
    from men 27–32
    need of competence in 2, 3, 4–5
    numbers of sexual partners 36–7
    older women 21–2
    as part of full history 10–11
    patient definition 6–7
    practising of 15–16
    sexual practices 37–8
    and specific problems 11
    timing of 8–12
    from women 17–26
    see also sexually transmissible disease (STD)
sexual rehabilitation in 97–8
sexually transmissible disease (STD) 67, 86–7, 111
    abnormal behaviours in 84–5
    confidentiality and 35
    history taking for 34–5, 40–1
    number of partners 36–7
    partner gender 37, 38–9
    patient attitudes to 69–76
    practitioner reactions to 77–8
    preventive health care 89
    and revealing sexuality 85–6
    and sexual practices 37–8
social drugs 102–3
STD see sexually transmissible disease
STD counselling 67, 86–7
    goals of 67–8, 77
    process in 68–9, 76
    psychological problems 76–7

T

therapist skills 44–7
trauma, from sexual practices 38
treatment compliance 39

V

vaginal intercourse 37

vaginismus 25–6
    treatments 61–2
venerophobia 71–3

W

women
    taking sexual history 17–26